◆◆◆◆◆◆◆◆◆◆◆◆◆◆◆◆◆◆◆◆◆◆◆◆◆◆◆◆◆◆◆◆◆◆

Xeroradiography: Uncalcified Breast Masses

◆◆◆◆◆◆◆◆◆◆◆◆◆◆◆◆◆◆◆◆◆◆◆◆◆◆◆◆◆◆◆◆◆

Xeroradiography: Uncalcified Breast Masses

By

JOHN N. WOLFE, M.D.

Chairman, Department of Radiology
Hutzel Hospital
Detroit, Michigan

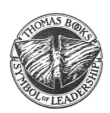

CHARLES C THOMAS · PUBLISHER
Springfield · Illinois · U.S.A.

Published and Distributed Throughout the World by
CHARLES C THOMAS • PUBLISHER
BANNERSTONE HOUSE
301-327 East Lawrence Avenue, Springfield, Illinois, U.S.A.

© *1977, by* CHARLES C THOMAS • PUBLISHER
ISBN 0-398-03504-0
Library of Congress Catalog Card Number: 75-33875

With THOMAS BOOKS *careful attention is given to all details of
manufacturing and design. It is the Publisher's desire to present books
that are satisfactory as to their physical qualities and artistic possibilities
and appropriate for their particular use.* THOMAS BOOKS *will be true
to those laws of quality that assure a good name and good will.*

Library of Congress Cataloging in Publication Data
Wolfe, John N
    Xeroradiography: uncalcified breast masses.

    Bibliography: p.
    Includes index.
1. Breast—Tumors—Diagnosis.   2. Breast—Radiography.
3. Xeroradiography.   I. Title.
RC280.B8W59   616.9'92'49   75-33875
ISBN 0-398-03504-0

Printed in the United States of America
P-4

I dedicate this book to my family and apologize for the time that it has taken me away from them.

Preface

A RADIOGRAPH OF THE BREAST will often exhibit a mass or masses in which there are no calcifications to aid in the diagnosis. This book presents information and graphic material to assist the radiologist in arriving at a reasonable differential diagnosis when confronted with such images.

The order of presentation proceeds from the obvious malignancies, characterized by a mass with a well-developed spiculated margin, to the more subtle circumscribed carcinomas, such as the medullary or colloid variety, and finally, to the most difficult of all, those that do not present as a well-defined mass but merely present as an area of increased density. The section will conclude with a presentation of some less common forms of malignancies. Following the section on malignancies, benign tumors will be considered in some detail.

The format of presentation will be illustrations of the classic type of pathology followed by examples of variations. Finally, cases will be shown in which one simply cannot arrive at a correct diagnosis. The reader should not be discouraged by this latter category as the vast majority of cases can be correctly diagnosed. It is considered advisable, however, to present the pitfalls also.

The fact that one must not only regard the radiographic features of the mass, but also its "environment" and the historical features will be stressed repeatedly throughout the text.

The advisability of reexamination after varying intervals will be discussed, a practice which is thought to be of great value, especially when one is rather confident the mass represents a cyst, hematoma or breast abscess.

The book is not intended to discuss completely the field of mammography, but it should be considered a supplement to standard textbooks on the subject.

Acknowledgments

A GREAT MANY PEOPLE contribute a tremendous amount of work toward writing a book. I want to express my sincere thanks to my office staff in particular Judy Brosch and Martine Jeza. Judy had the job of typing and re-typing the numerous manuscripts. Martine was constantly badgered to find specific case examples and to organize photographic material.

Without the cooperation of the Mammography Department staff, the quality of the illustrations could not have been achieved. I am indebted to Cornelia Steiman and all of her coworkers for affording me good images with which to work.

Elisa Petrini very attentively went over the text, rewriting much of it from the standpoint of sentence structure and punctuation. She has done, I believe, a good job.

I want to thank especially William Loranger, Ph.D. of the Xerox Corporation for the very early critique of the text. Doctor Loranger is the head of the Education Department of the Xeroradiography Program at Xerox, a close coworker and good friend of mine. His suggestions for revisions helped the text take shape.

I want to thank Mr. John Kroll for his usual good reproductions.

J.N.W.

Contents

◆◆

Xeroradiography: Uncalcified Breast Masses

◆◆

Chapter I

Introduction

UNCALCIFIED BREAST MASSES constitute a problem in differential diagnosis. Simply stated, the vast majority of them represent benign lesions; a very small percentage are carcinomas. A conception of the ratio of benign to malignant can be gained by realizing that slightly less than two in 100 discrete, noncalcified breast masses represent carcinomas.

Stated differently, slightly less than 50 percent of breast carcinomas present radiographically as masses without calcifications. Within this group of carcinomas without calcifications is a small number which are very discrete masses. These include those of the medullary or colloid variety. The question is, how does one find the small number of breast cancers within a large group of discrete tumors, nearly all of which are benign. As will be shown, every bit of information from the history, physical findings and radiographic observations must be used in arriving at a reasonable diagnosis.

A secondary area of interest is found in distinguishing between the types of various benign tumors. That is to say, is the mass a cyst, fibroadenoma, papilloma, hematoma, etc.? This may seem to be a relatively unimportant exercise as anyone would be happy to simply differentiate the benign from the malignant. It is interesting, however, to be able to be definite and correct in the diagnosis of the benign tumors, and it is possible, in many instances, to do this with a high degree of accuracy. There is some importance in determining if the mass represents a cyst, because aspiration of a cyst's contents can often be the definitive treatment.

The problem will be discussed in an orderly sequence of subjects with appropriate illustrations. Hopefully, the end result will be that one can be confident in the diagnosis of a vast majority of these tumors as either benign or malignant. One should realize that there are a small number of cases where it is impossible to have a firm opinion of benign or malignant disease, and the problem of what to recommend in these cases will be discussed. Generally, if one thinks it is a cyst, aspiration can be recommended. If the strongest opinion is for fibroadenoma, then periodic reexamination can be suggested, if the surgeon does not care to remove it. Each case has to be individualized as to the recommendation made.

It should be stressed, however, that one has to be extremely careful that the radiographic report does not discourage biopsy. The physical findings of the experienced examiner play a great role in the determination of whether or not the patient is going to have an excision biopsy. The report should be so constructed, however, that the radiologist gives his best opinion. If his best opinion is for benign disease, then that should be stated firmly. The examining physician is the one who makes the decision whether to biopsy or not, and he must be aware of the limitations as well as the positive aspects of the radiographic examination.

Chapter II

Carcinomas

THE DISCUSSION of the breast carcinoma which is not accompanied by calcifications will be divided into four parts, each of which corresponds to a particular type of carcinoma: (1) scirrhous, (2) nodular, (3) sharply circumscribed, and (4) noncircumscribed.

The key factors to consider in diagnosis concern the overall appearance of the mass, but especially its margins; its "environment," e.g. if there is a prominent duct pattern, then all masses are more suspect for carcinoma than otherwise; the historical features including the patient's age, and whether or not the mass that represents the carcinoma is palpable. Additional information such as skin retraction, pain, enlarged axillary lymph nodes, etc. is used when available.

SCIRRHOUS CARCINOMA

The term, *scirrhous carcinoma,* is used by the radiologist to connote a definable mass with a spiculated margin. It indicates that there is a considerable amount of connective tissue hyperplasia associated with the neoplasm. It is of passing interest that the spicules themselves may be composed solely of connective tissue or at times, a combination of connective tissue invaded by tumor cells. These spicules are characteristically short, usually from 2 to 10 millimeters in length but have been observed to be as long as 3 to 4 centimeters. They often extend to the skin and, in so doing, will produce retraction. (Figs. 1, 2, 3, 4, 5)

The scirrhous variety is the most common of the uncalcified breast cancers. It is the easiest to recognize and leads to the greatest accuracy in diagnosis. It is very rare to see a well-developed mass with a spiculated border and have the pathologist report that it is not a carcinoma. The usual cause for this is sclerosing adenosis or, rarely, other tumors such as fibroadenoma or fat necrosis.

If the observations made from the mammogram were such as to permit a firm diagnosis of carcinoma and the pathologist states a carcinoma is not present, the specimen should be radiographed. Failing to find an unobserved mass there, the radiologist should recommend that the patient be reexamined at some future date to ensure that the mass was indeed removed.

NODULAR FORM

This type of tumor is less common than the scirrhous variety. The carcinoma is characterized as a fairly well-limited mass with definable margins and no spiculation. Close inspection of it should reveal a faintly to rather well-pronounced nodular border. These tumors are often medullary carcinomas or simply carcinomas without a great deal of connective tissue hyperplasia. (Figs. 6, 7, 8, 9, 10, 11)

Nodular tumors tend to grow rather slowly. When their growth is observed over a period of time, what is most prominent on the interval examination is that they become more obviously malignant. That is to say, the faint nodularity present early in the stage of disease becomes more obvious. Spiculation may also develop along a segment of the margin. (Figs. 12, 13) Experience in observing the growth of these nodular carcinomas is limited, but what has been seen has been consistent.

It is very important to discuss the palpability of carcinomas at this point. When one is dealing with a scirrhous carcinoma with considerable connective tissue hyperplasia, the tumor will typically feel twice as large as it appears on the image. The medullary variety of carcinoma is a rather soft tumor without connective tissue hyperplasia, so that a medullary tumor as large as 2 centimeters could very easily escape detection by physical examination. One must not use the rule that, if it is

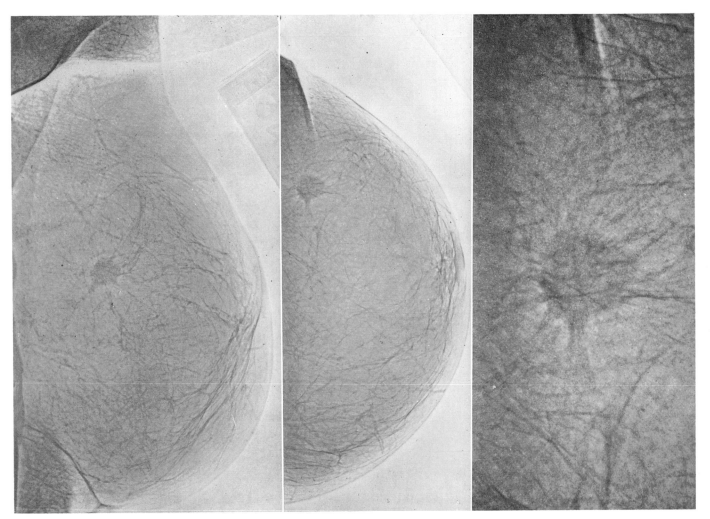

Figure 1.

HISTORY: A sixty-three-year-old, gravida 3 woman had had reduction mammoplasties on both breasts six years before examination. She complained of pain in both breasts and indentation of the skin on the left side below the level of the nipple.

RADIOGRAPHIC OBSERVATIONS: The mass with the spiculated margin was observed in the upper axillary quadrant of the left breast.

IMPRESSION: Scirrhous carcinoma.

HISTOPATHOLOGY: Carcinoma of the left breast.

DISCUSSION: The case is rather straightforward. The facts that the mass was nonpalpable, caused retraction and had an irregular margin produced by spiculation lead to a firm impression of carcinoma.

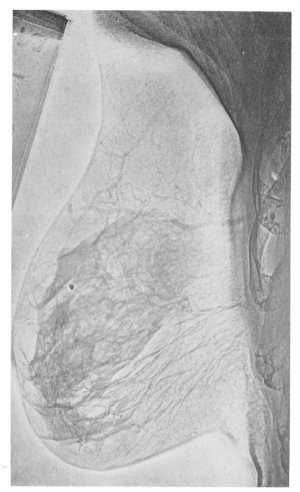
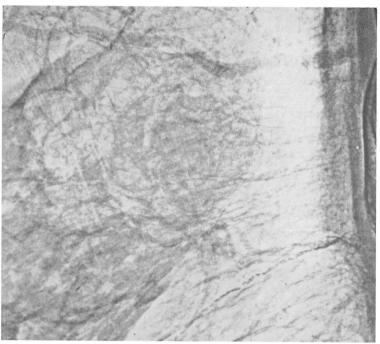

Figure 2.

HISTORY: A seventy-year-old, gravida 2 woman had slight thickening palpable in both breasts and no evidence of malignant disease from the physical examination. There are two studies separated by one year.

RADIOGRAPHIC OBSERVATIONS: (A, B) The breast was noted to be involved very severely with dysplasia and some element of a prominent duct pattern. Nothing was seen to suggest a carcinoma.

(C, D) One year later a spiculated density containing multiple small calcifications was observed. The spicules were very long, some measuring 2 to 4 cms.

IMPRESSION: (A, B) No evidence of carcinoma. (C, D) Strong radiographic evidence of carcinoma.

HISTOPATHOLOGY: Carcinoma of the breast with no metastatic disease to the axilla.

DISCUSSION: The case illustrates the difficulty of identifying some cancers even in retrospect. No carcinoma is evidenced on the first examination, even in the area shown to be malignant in Figure 2 C.

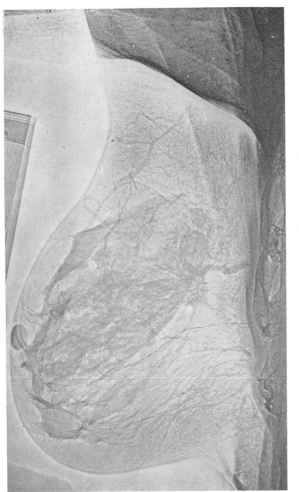
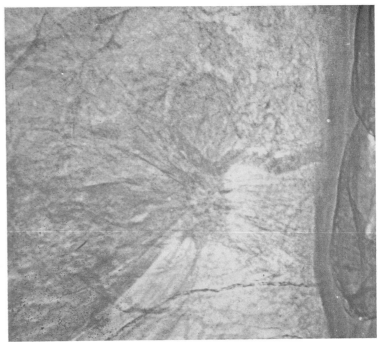

Figure 2 C-D *(Continued)*

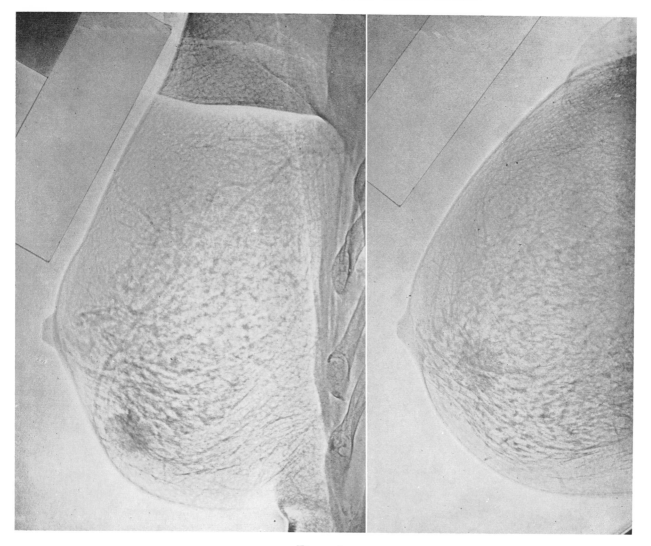

Figure 3.

HISTORY: A sixty-six-year old, gravida 1 woman discovered a mass in her left breast which on physical examination appeared to represent a carcinoma.

RADIOGRAPHIC OBSERVATIONS: A bilateral symmetrical prominent duct pattern of moderate severity was noted. The mass was readily observed. On close inspection one can see that it has a very irregular margin with faint spiculation.

IMPRESSION: Strong impression of scirrhous carcinoma.

HISTOPATHOLOGY: Scirrhous carcinoma.

DISCUSSION: The case does not appear to pose any particular problem especially in view of the spiculated margin of the mass. That, together with the prominent duct pattern, should lead one into a firm diagnosis of carcinoma.

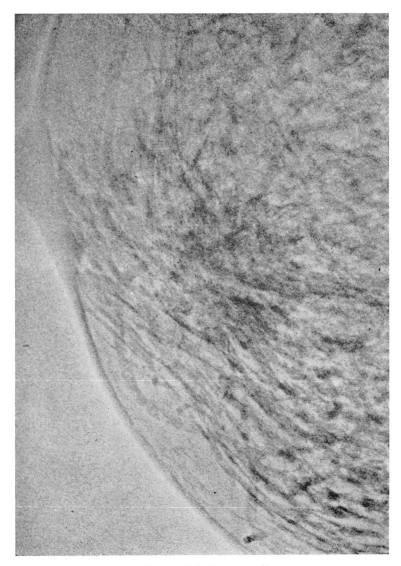

Figure 3 C *(Continued)*

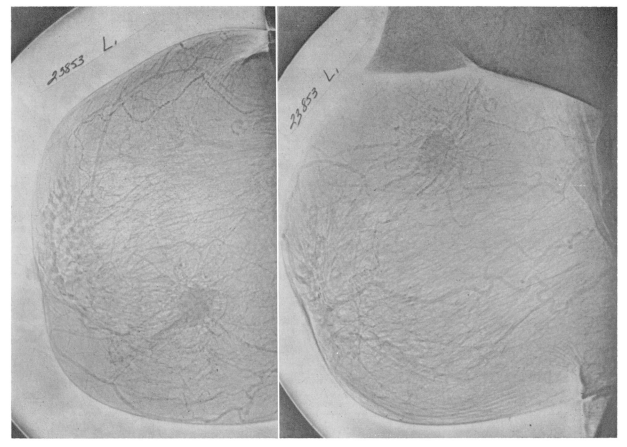

Figure 4.

HISTORY: An eighty-four-year-old, gravida 6 woman had had a right mastectomy thirty-five years before this study of the left breast. On self-examination she discovered a mass. The clinical impression was carcinoma.

RADIOGRAPHIC OBSERVATIONS: A moderate degree of prominent duct pattern was noted in the subareolar area. A mass in the upper quadrant was readily observed and noted to have a very irregular margin to it.

IMPRESSION: Carcinoma.

HISTOPATHOLOGY: Carcinoma.

DISCUSSION: The case does not pose any particular problem in diagnosis because of the faint spiculation around the margin of the mass.

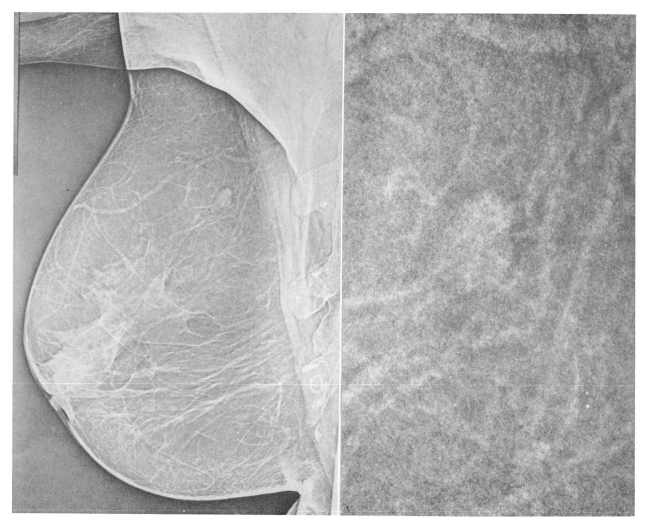

Figure 5.

HISTORY: A seventy-one-year-old, gravida 2 woman noted an inverted nipple and redness just above the nipple on the left side of short duration.

RADIOGRAPHIC OBSERVATIONS: The dysplasia on the left side was noted to be a little more severe as compared to the right. No obvious explanation was seen for the inverted nipple.

The most interesting finding was the small mass located high in the upper axillary quadrant. It was noted to have slightly irregular margins.

IMPRESSION: Suspicion of carcinoma of the left breast.

HISTOPATHOLOGY: Adenocarcinoma.

DISCUSSION: The differential diagnosis in this case would rest between an intramammary lymph node, other benign tumor and carcinoma. It was felt that perhaps it represented a carcinoma because of a slight irregularity of its margin. It was unilateral and, therefore, intramammary lymph node was discounted.

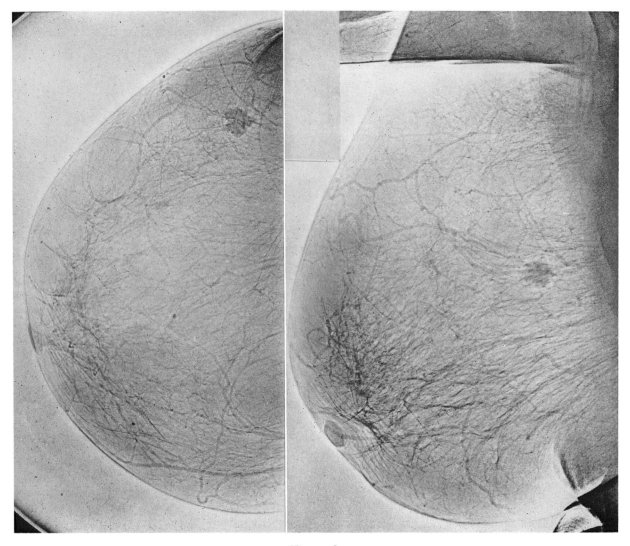

Figure 6.

HISTORY: A seventy-six-year-old, gravida 18 woman complained of pain in both breasts, with no abnormality palpable.

RADIOGRAPHIC OBSERVATIONS: Both breasts were noted to be involved with slight degrees of a prominent duct pattern in the anterior third. An irregular mass in the axillary portion of the left breast was identified and it was observed that its margin was very nodular.

IMPRESSION: Carcinoma.

HISTOPATHOLOGY: Carcinoma.

DISCUSSION: There should be no problem when one regards the tumor itself. Its border is extremely irregular being finely nodular. It is unusual for a woman who has had so many children to have a breast cancer. It is also unusual for such a woman to have a prominent duct pattern even to the minor degree observed. Probably the carcinoma and the prominent duct pattern go hand-in-hand.

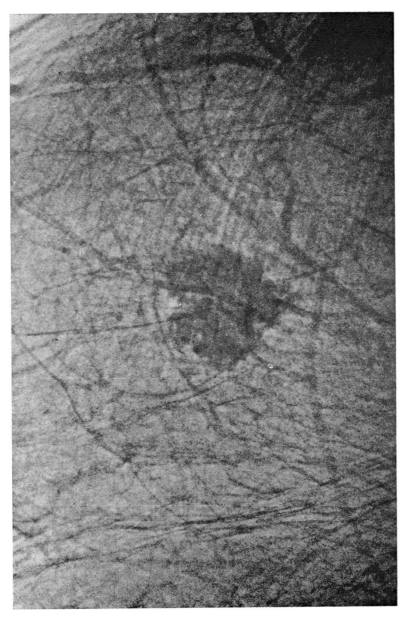

Figure 6 C *(Continued)*

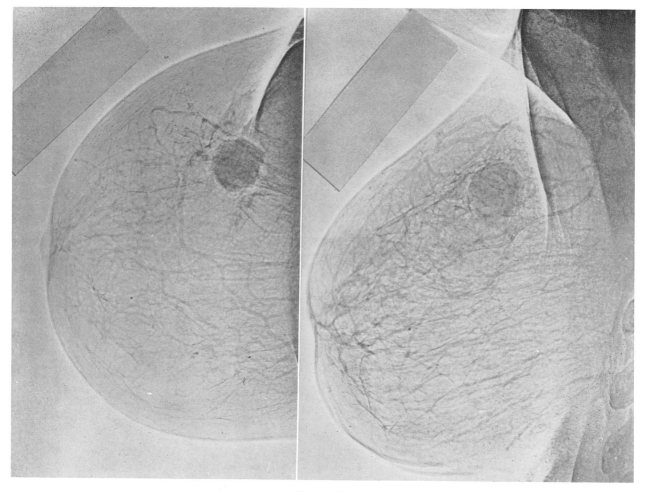

Figure 7.

HISTORY: A sixty-five-year-old, gravida 4 woman discovered a mass in the upper portion of her left breast. The clinical impression was indeterminate.

RADIOGRAPHIC OBSERVATIONS: The mass was apparent. The important observation concerned its wall and close inspection revealed definite nodularity. At no point was there a sharp border.

IMPRESSION: Medullary carcinoma.

HISTOPATHOLOGY: Medullary carcinoma.

DISCUSSION: One would expect to be right in this diagnosis at least 50 percent of the time. The radiographic impression should be rather firm because of the definite nodularity of the wall of the mass. The report should be worded in a way that would encourage the surgeon to biopsy.

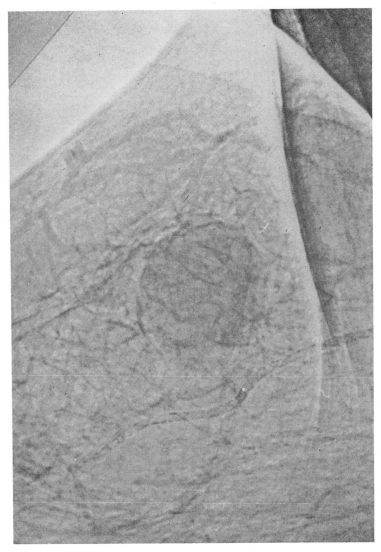

Figure 7 C *(Continued)*

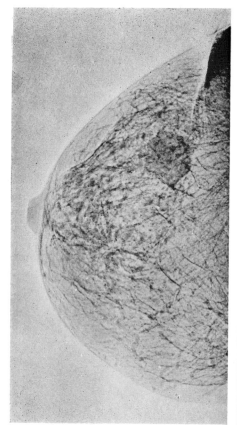
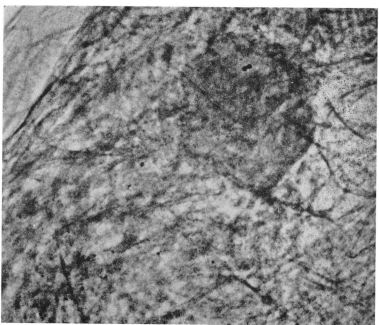

Figure 8.

HISTORY: A seventy-six-year-old woman had palpable abnormalities in both breasts. The changes were much more prominent on the left side and there was some suspicion for carcinoma from the physical examination.

RADIOGRAPHIC OBSERVATIONS: The circumscribed mass in the left breast was very apparent. Close inspection reveals its margin to be indistinct and there is one area which is somewhat nodular. Also noted is the associated prominent duct pattern. Of greater importance was the stellate density seen in the medial quadrant of the same breast containing several small calcifications.

IMPRESSION: Strong radiographic impression of two carcinomas of the left breast.

HISTOPATHOLOGY: Two carcinomas, the circumscribed one representing a medullary variety and the spiculated density representing a scirrhous carcinoma.

DISCUSSION: Simultaneous, multiple carcinomas of the breast are found in about 14 percent of cases. The somewhat discrete mass was strongly suspected for a medullary carcinoma because of its nodular margin. This criterion alone, however, affords only about 50 percent accuracy in diagnosis. The spiculated density, of course, leads to a firm impression of carcinoma with confirmation expected at least 90 percent of the time.

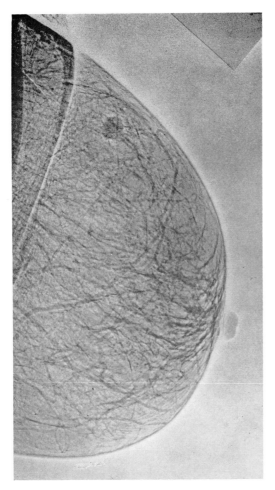
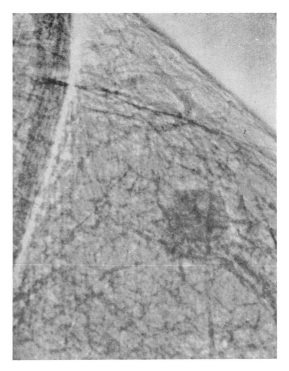

Figure 9.

HISTORY: A sixty-five-year-old, gravida 1 woman had slight thickening palpable in the axillary half of the right breast and a clinical impression of benign disease.

RADIOGRAPHIC OBSERVATIONS: The breast was observed to be involved with a slight degree of prominent duct pattern, not more than one would expect in a sixty-five-year-old, gravida 1 woman. The 9 millimeter mass was readily identified and its indistinct margin was noted.

IMPRESSION: Carcinoma, right breast.

HISTOPATHOLOGY: Carcinoma.

DISCUSSION: Despite the small size of the tumor, the very definite irregularity of its contours can be established. This evidence of malignancy leads to correct diagnosis about 50 percent of the time.

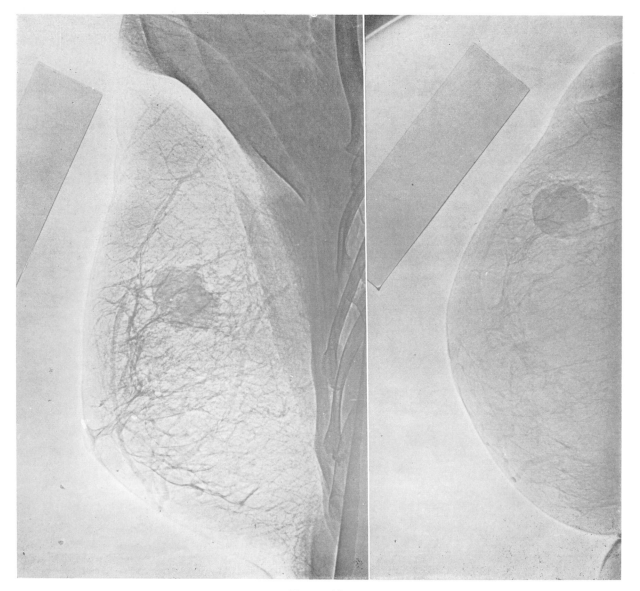

Figure 10.

HISTORY: A fifty-seven-year-old, gravida 2 woman injured her breast one month before this examination. On palpating the breast, she discovered a mass at the site of the injury in the upper axillary quadrant.

RADIOGRAPHIC OBSERVATIONS: The mass in the upper portion of the breast was readily identified. Close inspection of its margin, especially in the lateral projection, revealed a very nodular appearance without any sharp segment. The breast was composed mainly of fat and, if the mass truly had a sharp margin, one would expect to be able to identify it.

IMPRESSION: Carcinoma of the left breast, probably medullary.

HISTOPATHOLOGY: Medullary carcinoma.

DISCUSSION: The differential diagnosis with a mass such as this would rest primarily between a medullary carcinoma and a hematoma. A medullary carcinoma could be favored because of the faint nodularity of the mass. A hematoma is more likely to be composed of multiple masses but, of course, this is not always true. If one wanted to

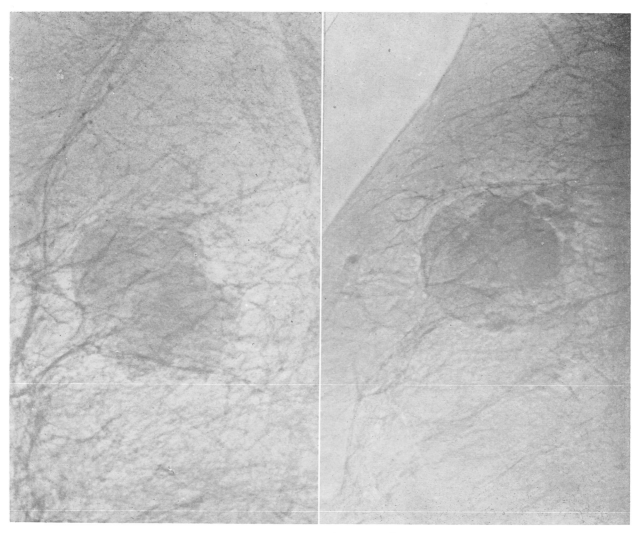

Figure 10 C-D *(Continued)*

be more certain of the diagnosis of benign or malignant disease, a reexamination after a short two- or three-week period would reveal some change if the mass represented a hematoma toward diminution in size, whereas one would not expect to see any change in the instance of carcinoma.

The radiographic features of the mass, however, are sufficient to warrant an immediate biopsy.

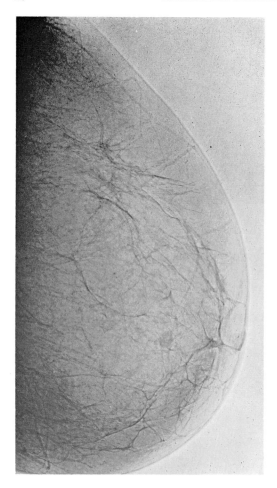
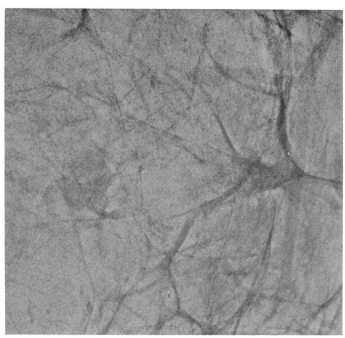

Figure 11.

HISTORY: A forty-nine-year-old, gravida 2 woman had a mass palpable in the lower quadrant of the left breast.

RADIOGRAPHIC OBSERVATIONS: The breasts were noted to be composed mainly of fat and no abnormality was seen on the left side. A faint 8 mm mass in the right breast was identified. Note that the margin was not sharp but somewhat nodular.

IMPRESSION: Carcinoma, right breast.

HISTOPATHOLOGY: Carcinoma.

DISCUSSION: This represents an occult carcinoma. In a case such as this, one would expect to be correct in the diagnosis of carcinoma probably 75 percent of the time. The errors would concern mainly fibroadenomas.

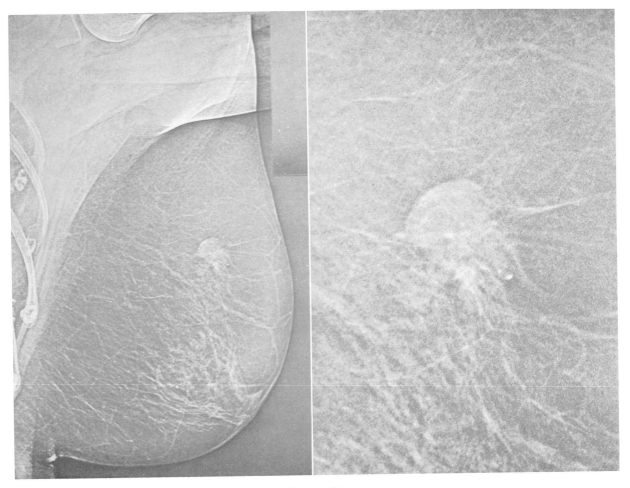

Figure 12.

HISTORY: A fifty-five-year-old, gravida 2 woman had a mass palpable in the breast and an indeterminate clinical impression.

RADIOGRAPHIC OBSERVATIONS: The mass was very apparent. It was noted that the posterior margin was rather sharp, but the anterior margin was very irregular.

IMPRESSION: Carcinoma.

HISTOPATHOLOGY: Carcinoma.

DISCUSSION: This is a fairly good demonstration of the tendency of a well-circum-scribed carcinoma to extend. Often, a segment of its margin represents a sharp line of demarcation between the mass and adjoining breast tissue, but along other portions of the border obvious evidence of carcinoma can be seen.

palpable, it is more likely to represent a carcinoma. As a matter of fact, fibroadenomas and cysts are probably more readily palpable than the typical medullary carcinoma. (Fig. 14)

Fibroadenomas will at times simulate the nodular form of carcinoma exactly, and it is impossible to avoid biopsy in such cases. Similarly, cysts will occasionally have nodular borders. One case of fat necrosis presenting as a solid tumor of nonfat density was diagnosed with a great deal of confidence as a nodular form of carcinoma.

SHARPLY CIRCUMSCRIBED FORM

This is one of the very difficult forms of carcinoma to diagnose. It represents only a very small number of the total malignancies, probably about 2 percent at most. An attempt must be made to differentiate these carcinomas, usually of the medullary or colloid variety, from the myriad number of benign tumors that could have an identical appearance. The margin of the tumor is the main area to examine, and it may vary from being gently lobular to extremely sharp. (Figs. 15, 16, 17, 18, 19, 20)

The well-circumscribed forms of carcinoma occur infrequently in young women, at least in the experience of this author. A well-circumscribed tumor in the woman below the age of thirty is nearly always a fibroadenoma. However, of the lobulated, uncalcified tumors in women above that age, although very likely to be fibroadenomas or cysts, a small number will be carcinomas. It is suggested, therefore, that extreme caution be used in the dictation of the radiographic report, and biopsy should not be discouraged. Depending on the circumstances, interval examination no sooner than three nor later than four months may be employed. The greatest value of the interval examination is in diagnosis of cysts because they fluctuate over short periods of time. This will be discussed more completely in the section on cysts.

This form of carcinoma can also be simulated by cysts. Therefore, when the bulk of the evidence indicates that the mass represents a cyst, aspiration of its contents can be a worthwhile diagnostic and therapeutic procedure and should be recommended. The possibility of failing to observe a carcinoma arising in a cyst by this maneuver is extremely slight. To begin with, carcinomas arising in the wall of a cyst are rarely seen. If there is a carcinoma, the cyst's contents frequently contain blood and can be stained for tumor cells. Finally, if there is a carcinoma arising in the wall of the cyst, it is likely that the fluid contents will reaccumulate in a very short period of time, usually four to six weeks. In the instance of the cyst, the contents are unlikely to recur in such a short period of time, if at all. One can also inject air into the cyst after aspiration and outline the contour of the inner wall.

NONCIRCUMSCRIBED MASSES

This type of carcinoma does not precisely fit into the general format of the presentations in this book because it does not form a discrete mass. It is included, however, to complete the presentation of types of carcinoma one may encounter which may not contain calcifications. (Figs. 21, 22)

There are certain aspects of noncircumscribed masses which are important and interesting to the radiologist. These carcinomas are the most difficult to identify because they do not form distinct masses and, when recognized, they are seen only as an area of increased density. In addition, such masses are typically rapid growing which one might suspect from their failure to form distinct masses or develop calcifications. They also are the type of carcinoma the radiologist is most likely to fail to observe, especially in the "dense" breast.

This tumor is the type that one identifies especially as areas of asymmetry. This is an important technic of interpretation. One should inspect both breasts and look for asymmetrical areas of added density. Fortunately, most of these asymmetrical areas represent merely benign abnormalities of the breast, such as adenosis. (Fig. 23)

This cancer is also prone to have extensive regional lymph node metastases when first discovered, either by radiographic means or physical examination. The carcinomas tend to occur in breasts which appear "active," that is, those containing a great amount of mammary dysplasia. When first seen, there are often stigmata of advanced disease, such as enlarged axillary lymph nodes and edema of the skin. In an early stage they can be rather limited in their extent of mass

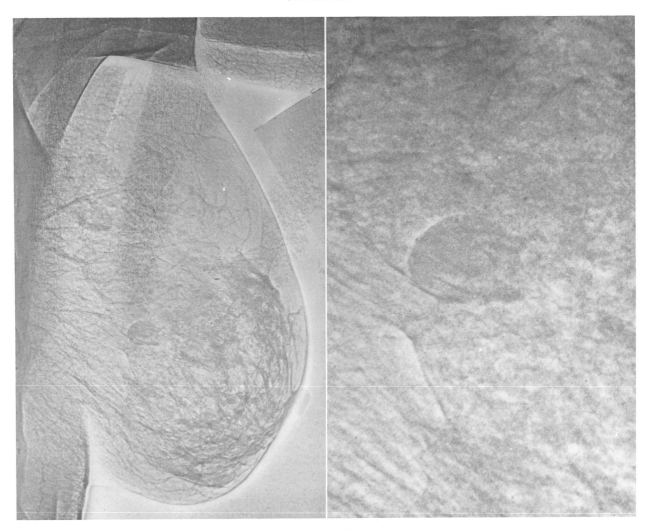

Figure 13.

HISTORY: A fifty-six-year-old gravida 3 woman has had numerous biopsies and cyst aspirations of both breasts in the past and now has bilateral palpable masses. The dominant mass is on the left, and an attempt to aspirate it was unsuccessful.

RADIOGRAPHIC OBSERVATIONS: Both breasts were noted to be involved with a prominent duct pattern and mammary dysplasia. The mass in the left breast was noted to have a very nodular margin, whereas the one on the right was sharply circumscribed.

IMPRESSION: Carcinoma, probably medullary, left breast.

HISTOPATHOLOGY: Carcinoma, left breast.

DISCUSSION: The case is a good example of bilateral involvement with masses and demonstrates the importance of examining each margin individually. The carcinoma has a very definite nodularity near the periphery. The calcifications were considered of no importance; several types were observed including fine punctate ones of adenosis and large granular calcifications probably the result of previous fibroadenomas.

It is of considerable interest that the patient had an examination six months before at which time masses were present in both breasts. The one representing the carcinoma changed by enlarging approximately 25 percent and, most important, its margin became very nodular.

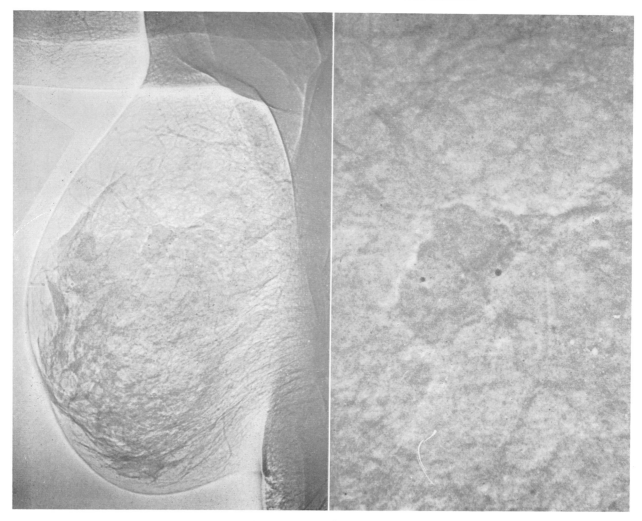

Figure 13 C-D *(Continued)*

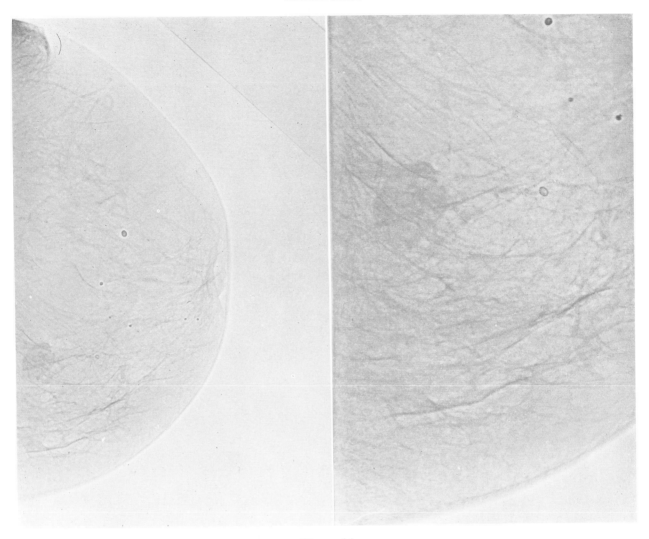

Figure 14.

HISTORY: A sixty-year-old, gravida 1 woman with a history of biopsy of the left breast twenty-five years before, discovered a mass in the lower portion of the right breast.

RADIOGRAPHIC OBSERVATIONS: The retracted nipple was identified, but that existed bilaterally, and was not considered significant. The mass was rather evident and, most important, its nodular border was observed. Calcifications were considered a result of retention of lactiferous material sometime in the past.

IMPRESSION: Carcinoma, right breast.

HISTOPATHOLOGY: Carcinoma.

DISCUSSION: The tumor was palpable. On the lateral projection (not shown) it was noted to be rather superficial near the inframammary fold. The nodular margin is the chief observation which permits the correct diagnosis of carcinoma. A small mass such as this, being readily palpable, is also significant.

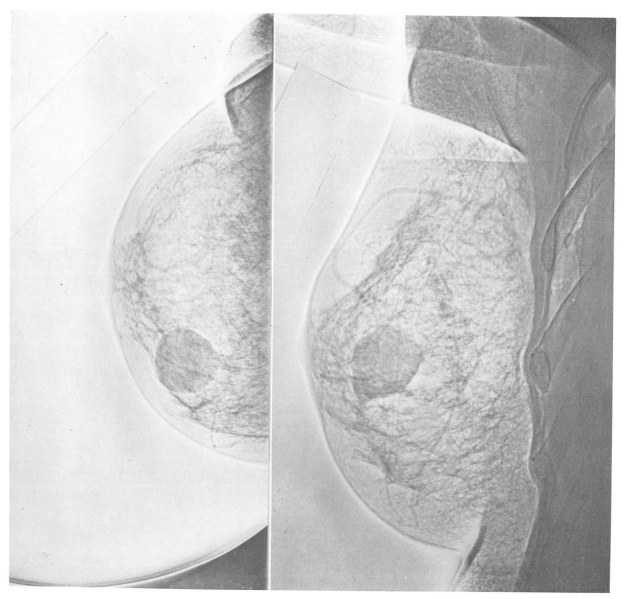

Figure 15.

HISTORY: A forty-eight-year-old, gravida 1 woman had a mass in the left breast and a history of two previous biopsies of the left breast.

RADIOGRAPHIC OBSERVATIONS: Both breasts were observed to be involved with a prominent duct pattern that seemed more severe than that usually observed in a forty-eight-year-old woman. A 2 cm mass was readily identified and its margin in the caudal projection was very sharp. In the lateral projection, however, one could detect some slight tapering at one end and very faint nodularity at the other.

IMPRESSION: Suspicion for medullary carcinoma of the breast.

HISTOPATHOLOGY: Medullary carcinoma.

DISCUSSION: This case is illustrative of the care with which one must interpret solitary masses in the presence of a prominent duct pattern and especially in women in the cancer-prone age group. It is believed the chances of this impression of car-

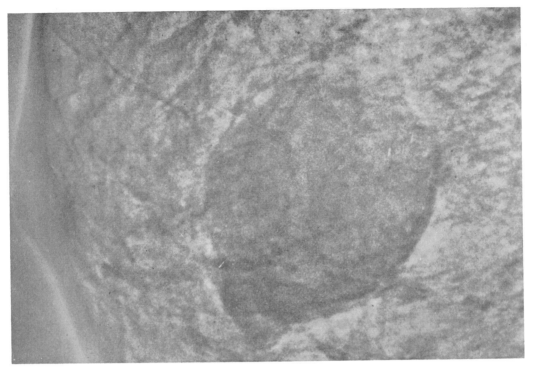

Figure 15 C *(Continued)*

cinoma being correct are less than 25 percent. It would have been much more likely to discover a cyst or, secondly, a fibroadenoma. A slight increased venous vascularity to the side with the tumor was also noted which added a little weight to the impression of carcinoma.

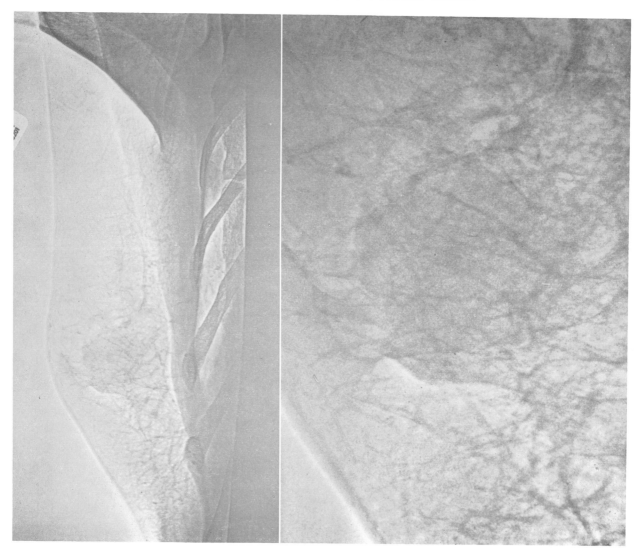

Figure 16.

HISTORY: A forty-nine-year-old, gravida 4 woman discovered a lump in her left breast and on physical examination it was thought to represent benign disease.

RADIOGRAPHIC OBSERVATIONS: The mass in the central portion of the breast was readily identified. Close inspection of the margins did not reveal a sharp segment in any portion, yet is was not a lobulated tumor like fibroadenoma. It was viewed with considerable suspicion for carcinoma.

IMPRESSION: Possible medullary carcinoma with a differential diagnosis of cyst.

HISTOPATHOLOGY: Medullary carcinoma.

DISCUSSION: Most masses located in the central portion of small breasts represent cysts. This was thought more likely to represent a medullary carcinoma because no segment of the wall of the mass is completely sharp. It was believed the likelihood of it representing a carcinoma was about 50 percent.

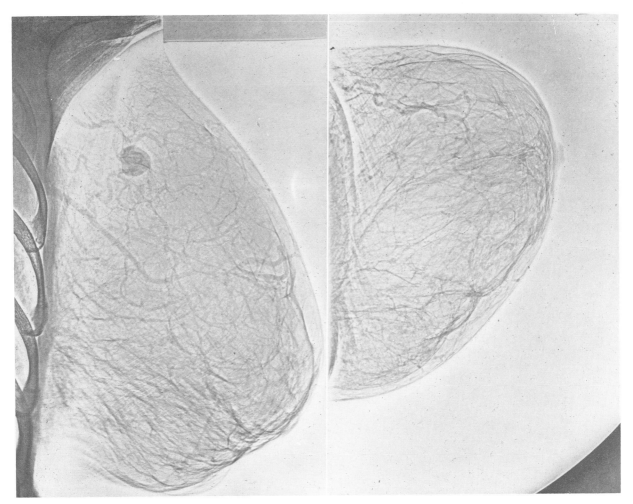

Figure 17.

HISTORY: A sixty-five-year-old, gravida 2 woman had a mass palpable in the upper axillary quadrant of the right breast and a clinical impression of benign disease.

RADIOGRAPHIC OBSERVATIONS: The mass in the right breast was rather sharply limited, but the margin, on close inspection, was not as perfectly clear-cut as one would expect a cyst or fibroadenoma to be. There was very slight indistinctness posteriorly. (The spiculated mass observed in the opposite breast was considered characteristic of carcinoma.)

IMPRESSION: Medullary carcinoma, right breast. Scirrhous carcinoma, left breast.

HISTOPATHOLOGY: Medullary carcinoma, right breast. Scirrhous carcinoma, left breast.

DISCUSSION: The indistinctness of the margin and the slight posterior irregularity make the mass suspicious for malignancy. Based on this evidence, its chances of representing a carcinoma are probably less than 50 percent. More likely it would represent a fibroadenoma and, as a second possibility, a cyst.

Although the mass is larger than the usual normal intramammary lymph node, it is not larger than an intramammary lymph node involved with metastatic neoplastic disease.

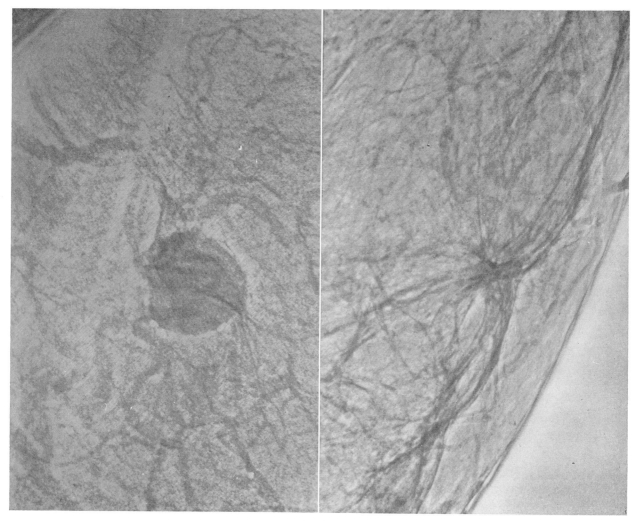

Figure 17 C *(Continued)*

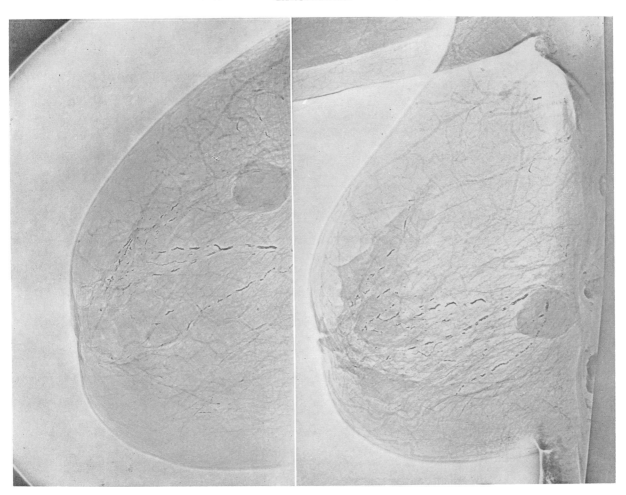

Figure 18.

HISTORY: A sixty-two-year-old woman had a mass palpable in the axillary quadrant of the left breast. The clinical impression was carcinoma.

RADIOGRAPHIC OBSERVATIONS: The breast was noted to be involved with a prominent duct pattern and there were calcifications typical for secretory disease and arteriosclerosis.

The mass was readily identified. It was noted not to have a completely sharp margin.

IMPRESSION: Carcinoma, probably medullary.

HISTOPATHOLOGY: Carcinoma.

DISCUSSION: The age of this patient, the associated prominent duct pattern and the indistinctness of the mass together with it being palpable, leads to a straightforward diagnosis of carcinoma of the breast. One would expect to be right about 75 percent of the time in diagnosis of a tumor such as this. It would not be too surprising if it represented a cyst.

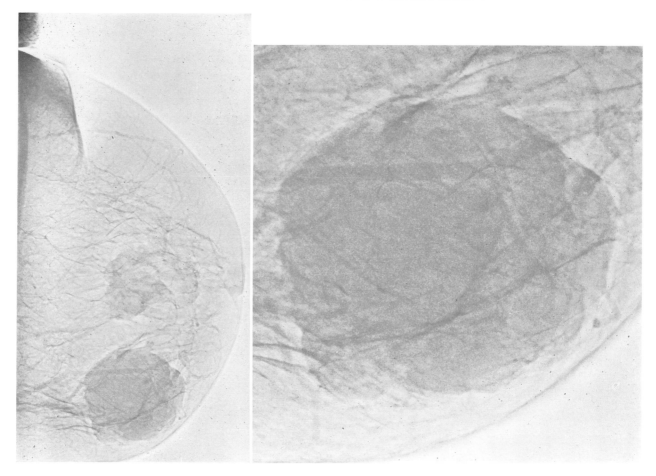

Figure 19.

HISTORY: A forty-four-year-old, gravida 6 woman discovered masses in both breasts and the clinical impression was indeterminate.

RADIOGRAPHIC OBSERVATIONS: The breast was noted to be composed mainly of fat with only a few duct-like structures in the anterior third. These changes were bilateral and symmetrical. Two masses were observed in the right breast. Note that the mass in the subareolar area was irregular with some spiculation around the periphery. The larger mass was fairly circumscribed, but it was definitely nodular toward its posterior margin.

IMPRESSION: Two carcinomas, right breast.

HISTOPATHOLOGY: Two carcinomas, right breast, the larger is medullary.

DISCUSSION: The larger mass, in the presence of the other more obvious carcinoma, is confidently regarded as a second primary. Considered alone, however, it is somewhat more difficult to identify. Its location, far to the medial aspect, makes its suspicious for malignancy, but masses like this often represent fibroadenomas. Its faintly nodular border appears to be the best clue to the correct diagnosis.

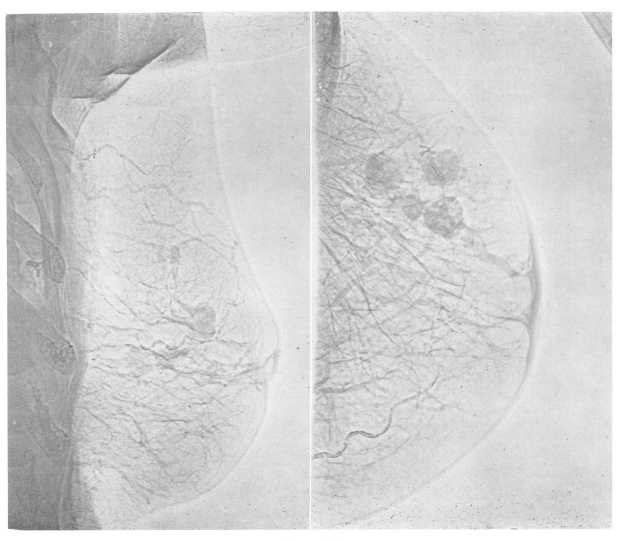

Figure 20.

HISTORY: An eighty-year-old, gravida 2 with a bloody nipple discharge from the right breast.

RADIOGRAPHIC OBSERVATIONS: The breasts were noted to be composed mainly of fat with only a few ducts in the subareolar areas. There were four readily identifiable masses. There was a large duct extending from the subareolar area to the region of the masses. The margins of the masses were noted to be somewhat lobular.

IMPRESSION: Multiple carcinomas, right breast with a differential diagnosis to include multiple papillomas.

HISTOPATHOLOGY: Multiple intraductal carcinomas.

DISCUSSION: Multiple, unilateral masses which occupy a relatively small area such as these should be considered rather strongly for carcinoma especially if nodularity of their margins can be demonstrated such as in this case. Papillomas can sometimes but rarely have an appearance such as this. One would not expect fibroadenomas to be so closely associated one with the other, nor would they be expected to be unilateral. Cysts could conceivably have an appearance such as this, but it would be an extremely unusual occurrence.

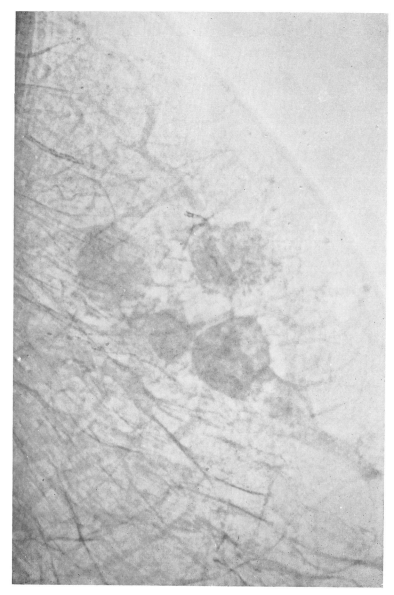

Figure 20 C *(Continued)*

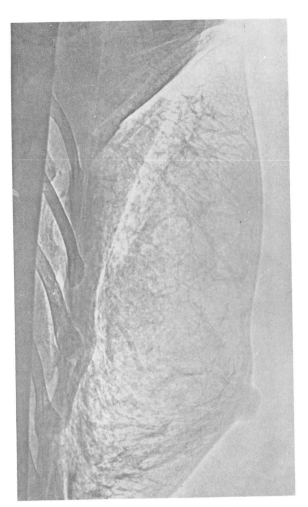 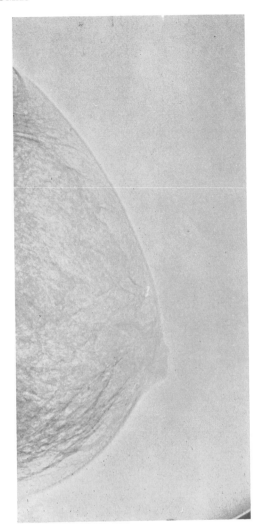

Figure 21.

HISTORY: A thirty-nine-year-old, gravida 2 woman appeared for an examination complaining of thickening in both breasts. The XR's at that time were interpreted as representing merely severe mammary dysplasia. The physical findings were those of benign disease.

She returned thirteen months later with a mass palpable in the right breast.

RADIOGRAPHIC OBSERVATIONS: The breasts were noted to be involved rather severely with dysplasia. A poorly limited mass, about 3 cms in diameter, could be located deep near the chest wall and slightly above the level of the nipple on the lateral projection. The features were thought to be those of a carcinoma and probably a rapidly growing type.

IMPRESSION: Carcinoma.

HISTOPATHOLOGY: Carcinoma with all levels of lymph nodes involved with metastases.

DISCUSSION: These are the most difficult tumors to diagnose by mammography and they are also the most rapidly growing. In the relatively short thirteen-month period, the physical and radiographic examinations went from no significant abnormality to an obvious carcinoma by both modalities.

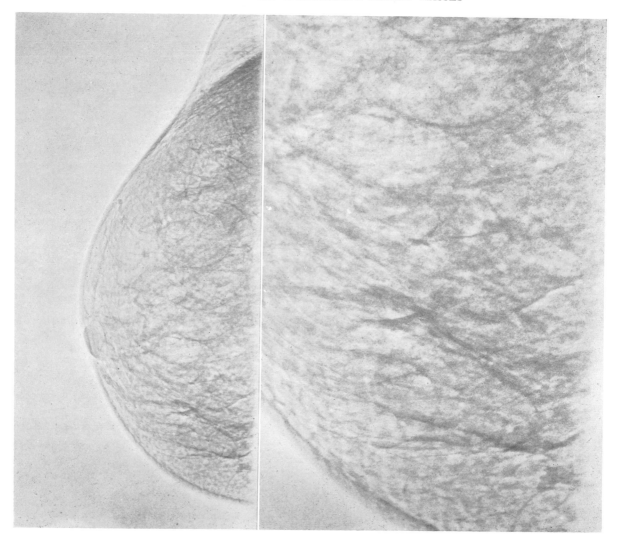

Figure 22.

HISTORY: A sixty-one-year-old, gravida 2 woman discovered an area of thickening in her right breast. The clinical impression was benign disease.

RADIOGRAPHIC OBSERVATIONS: The breasts were involved rather symmetrically with a prominent duct pattern of moderate severity. The irregular mass-like density was observed. No sharp margin could be identified and there were no calcifications.

IMPRESSION: Carcinoma.

HISTOPATHOLOGY: Carcinoma.

DISCUSSION: The case appears straightforward. The mass is apparent. It does not have a sharp margin to it. There is an associated prominent duct pattern. In this age group and with these observations, one certainly has to have a firm opinion of malignancy. Carcinomas such as this are considered rapidly growing when they do not form well-defined spiculations and such was the case here, multiple lymph nodes were involved with metastases.

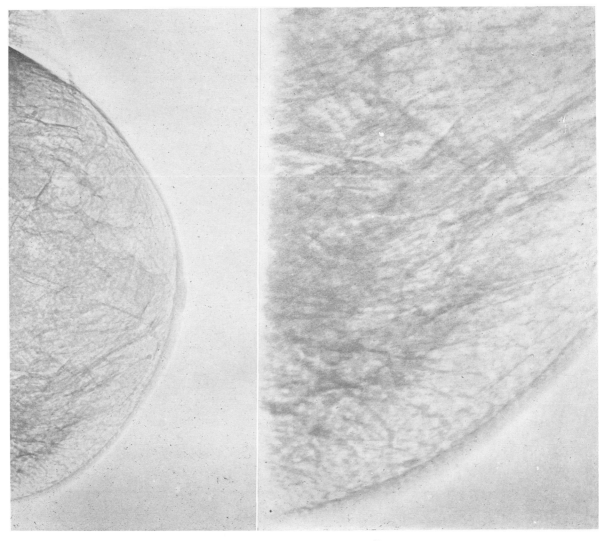

Figure 22 C-D *(Continued)*

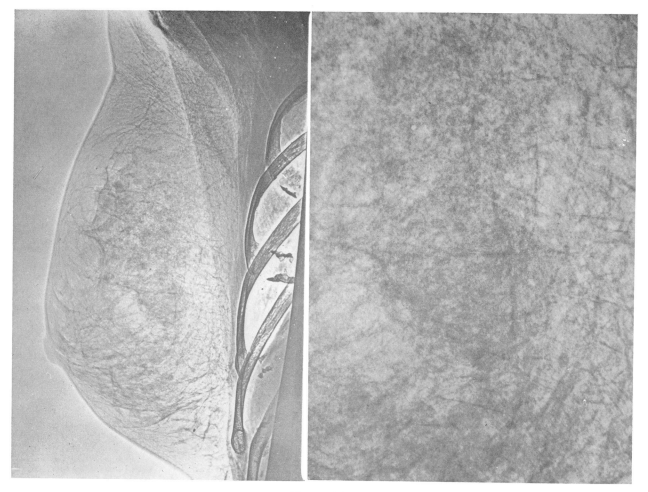

Figure 23.

HISTORY: A forty-five-year-old, gravida 1 woman had palpable masses in both breasts and a clinical impression of benign disease.

RADIOGRAPHIC OBSERVATIONS: A somewhat mass-like area of increased density was noted in the midportion of the left breast. The margin of the mass was irregular. No tumor calcification could be identified.

IMPRESSION: The mass was regarded with suspicion for a rapidly growing carcinoma.

HISTOPATHOLOGY: Adenosis.

DISCUSSION: This represents a very difficult case for differential diagnosis. Some rapidly growing carcinomas present only as asymmetrical areas of increased density which do not form distinct masses. They are not usually accompanied by calcifications. Adenosis presents as a similar abnormality. One would expect to be right in the diagnosis of carcinoma in these instances only about 20 percent of the time.

formation, but it is believed that as the tumors progress, they frequently evolve into the diffuse type of carcinoma with widespread involvement. (Fig. 24)

It is important to point out that there are other diagnostic criteria for the identification of breast carcinoma which do not fit into this discussion of uncalcified breast masses. Some are identified chiefly by distortion of the architectural pattern, calcific pattern, skin edema, skin retraction and increased vascularity. As stated in the Preface, no attempt is being made to relate all aspects of breast disease. Rather, the attempt here is to present a differential diagnosis of discrete breast masses not associated with calcifications.

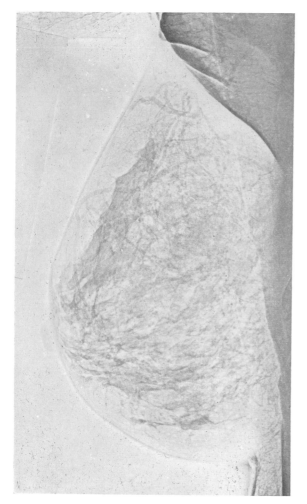 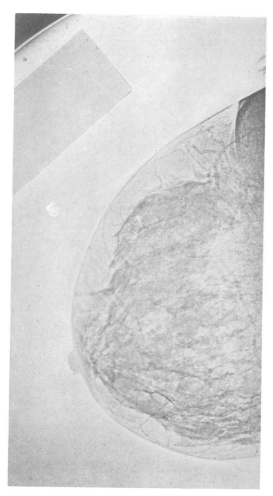

Figure 24.

HISTORY: A forty-five-year-old, gravida 1 woman came for a routine first examination with slight thickening palpable in the upper quadrants of both breasts. There are two examinations, separated by approximately eighteen months.

RADIOGRAPHIC OBSERVATIONS: On the first study the breasts were symmetrically involved with a severe prominent duct pattern. No abnormality to suggest a carcinoma could be observed (A).

On the second examination, rather clear-cut signs of carcinoma were identified: a somewhat diffuse mass in the upper axillary quadrant and marked edema of the skin and areola (B).

IMPRESSION: Carcinoma.

HISTOPATHOLOGY: Carcinoma with multiple lymph nodes involved with metastases.

DISCUSSION: This is an example of a rapidly growing carcinoma. On the first study, one notes the moderately severe dysplasia with a prominent duct pattern which is some indication that she is at a higher risk for breast cancer development. The second study, of course, reveals clearly the rapidly growing neoplasm.

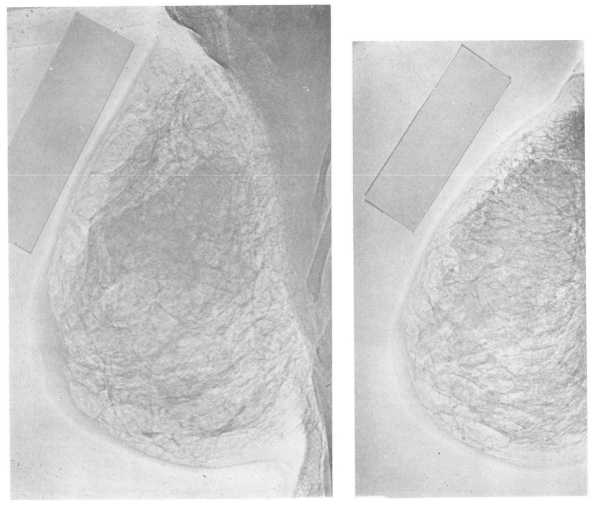

Figure 24 C-D *(Continued)*

Chapter III

Sarcomas

SARCOMAS OF THE BREAST are rare, accounting for only about 0.5 percent of all breast malignancies. When first seen, they are usually in an advanced state. The most common sarcomas are the cystosarcoma phylloides.

CYSTOSARCOMA PHYLLOIDES

Cystosarcoma phylloides is a rare form of sarcoma, and in an advanced stage, it usually can be recognized readily when considered in conjunction with the history and physical findings. As a rule, it is multilobulated and very large. There is a history of rapid growth and on physical examination the mass has a cystic consistency. Frequently there is a discernible increased venous vascularity that one can see by inspection of the skin of the breast or the mammogram. (Fig. 25)

Cystosarcomas, when detected early, have the appearance of a fibroadenoma. This is not surprising when one considers that insofar as the tissues are concerned, fibroadenomas and cystosarcomas have exactly the same components except that in the latter the connective tissue component is sarcomatous.

There are many mistakes made in calling masses within the breast cystosarcoma phylloides. In reality, many are not. The most common error results from giant fibroadenomas in adults. Errors have also been made in the instance of very large abscesses, which at times can be multilobulated. Examples of these can be found in the appropriate sections on those subjects. (Fig. 26)

ANGIOSARCOMA

One case of angiosarcoma has been seen, and it was thought to be a cystosarcoma from its radiographic features. The important observations included a history of a rapidly growing, unilateral mass which was extremely hard to palpation and was accompanied by observable increased superficial venous vascularity. A form of sarcoma other than cystosarcoma should have been suspected because of the physical finding of the "rock-hard" mass. The cystosarcoma usually has a cystic consistency. (Fig. 27)

A reasonable differential diagnosis between carcinoma and sarcoma was not difficult because carcinomas usually do not grow as rapidly as was observed in the case of the angiosarcoma where there was only a two-month history from a normal breast to one with a mass 8 centimeters in diameter.

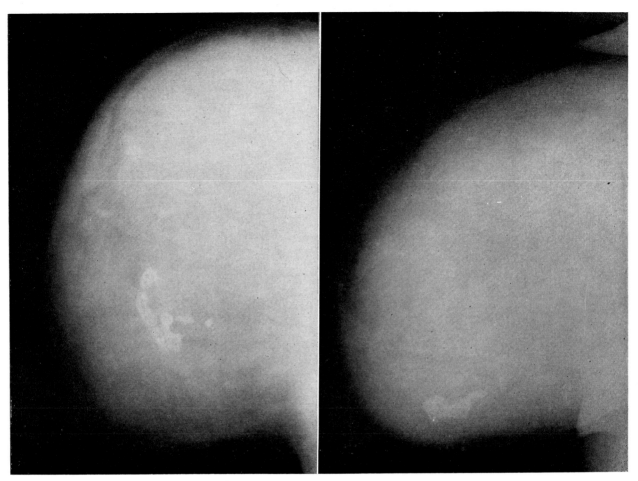

Figure 25.

HISTORY: The patient is a fifty-five-year-old woman who had a huge mass palpable in the breast of three year's duration accompanied by thickening of the skin.

RADIOGRAPHIC OBSERVATIONS: The very large, somewhat homogeneous mass was identified together with edema of the skin. The unusual form of calcification was also noted.

RADIOGRAPHIC IMPRESSION: Cystosarcoma phylloides.

HISTOPATHOLOGY: Cystosarcoma.

DISCUSSION: Considering the history, physical findings and radiographic observations, apart from the calcifications, the most likely radiographic impression would be cystosarcoma phylloides. One would not expect to be correct in this impression more than 50 percent of the time. Often, such a mass represents simply a giant fibroadenoma, or rarely, a papilloma or some other form of sarcoma such as reticulum cell sarcoma.

The calcifications are somewhat characteristic of cystosarcoma phylloides.

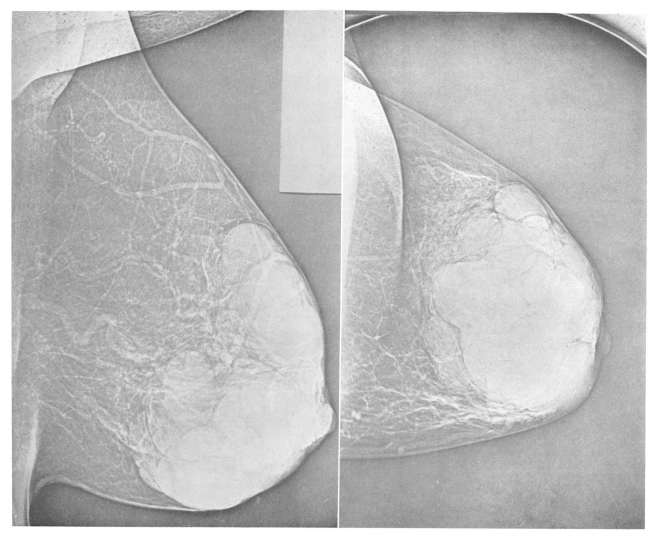

Figure 26.

HISTORY: A forty-four-year-old, gravida 7 woman had a biopsy of the right breast eleven years before at which time multiple masses were removed. She now complains that the right breast is enlarging and that there is a mass in the subareolar area.

RADIOGRAPHIC OBSERVATIONS: The breasts were noted to be composed mainly of fat. The vascularity to the right side appeared to have increased tremendously with veins being fully three times greater in diameter than those in the left breast. The markedly lobulated mass in the subareolar area was very evident, and it had many components. The margins of each component appeared sharp and distinct. No calcifications were noted.

The history of prior removal of multiple masses from the right breast was considered significant.

IMPRESSION: Cystosarcoma phylloides.

HISTOPATHOLOGY: Cystosarcoma phylloides, benign. Some would regard this merely as a fibroadenoma or giant fibroadenoma.

DISCUSSION: The marked lobularity of the mass, together with the significantly increased vascularity, point to a diagnosis of a malignant tumor and in this case, of course, a cystosarcoma. Cysts do not have a propensity to be subareolar and markedly lobulated as this tumor does, and the possibility that it represents a simple carcinoma is very slight.

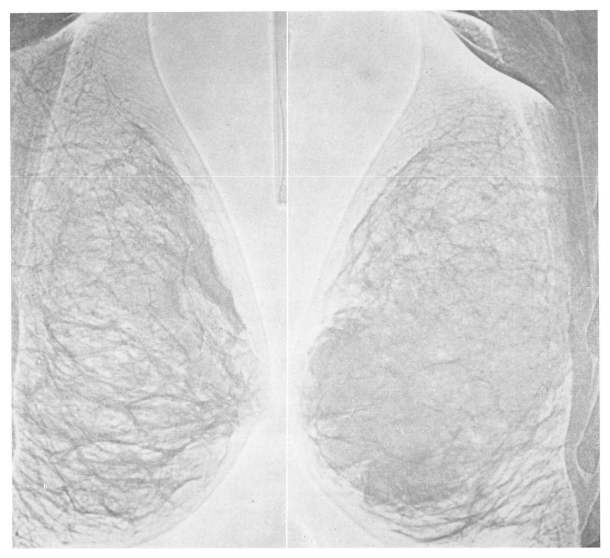

Figure 27.

HISTORY: A twenty-nine-year-old, nulliparous woman noted an enlargement of the right breast of three month's duration. The enlargement was mass-like and extremely hard to palpation. There was some pain.

RADIOGRAPHIC OBSERVATIONS: (A) normal side, (B) abnormal side. The breasts were considered essentially normal except for the mass-like area of increased density in the central portion which on the axillary view showed it to be in the lateral half. It appeared to be somewhat multilobulated, but not sharply limited. There was increased venous vascularity.

IMPRESSION: Cystosarcoma phylloides.

HISTOPATHOLOGY: Angiosarcoma.

DISCUSSION: If one considers the radiographic observations in light of the history of this patient, a diagnosis of benign or ordinary malignant disease of the breast should not be considered. The time span for a carcinoma is much too short. Also, extremely large carcinomas such as this are somewhat unusual in young women. Rapidly-growing carcinomas in young women do not tend to form obvious masses.

The most logical conclusion would be an unusual abnormality of the breast, and cysto-sarcoma or some form of sarcoma would be the most likely. One feature against cystosarcoma is that the mass was extremely hard to palpation, and cystosarcomas generally have a cystic feel and are not hard.

Chapter IV

Malignancies Involving the Reticuloendothelial System

THE MOST FREQUENT observation made from the mammogram in patients with neoplasm of the reticuloendothelial system concerns enlarged axillary lymph nodes. A few can be seen, however, where there are discrete masses within the breast.

LYMPHOMA

Lymphoma of the breast usually presents itself as a diffuse, nonlimited, mass-like area of increased density and there is evidence of the disease elsewhere in the body. One case, characterized by discrete, uncalcified masses, has been seen and was mistakenly diagnosed as a possible bilateral carcinoma. As one can see in the illustration, the masses, although fairly well defined, do not have perfectly sharp margins and, for that reason, they were suspected of being carcinomas. The patient did not have other evidence of lymphoma at the time of breast surgery. (Fig. 28)

RETICULUM CELL SARCOMA

Several cases of reticulum cell sarcoma have been observed and, more than anything else, their characteristics were those of a very rapidly growing mass. The masses appeared to be rather well-limited and calcifications were not observed in association with them. The involvement of the breast was always in association with generalized disease. (Fig. 29)

PLASMACYTOMA

Plasmacytomas usually have the configuration of fibroadenomas. That is to say, they are sharply circumscribed tumors without calcifications. At times they are lobulated. Although most of the cases have been unilateral, some bilateral ones have been observed. (Fig. 30)

Without the proper history of multiple myeloma, the practice has been to identify them always as being benign tumors, most likely fibroadenomas. If one has the knowledge that the patient has multiple myeloma, then a more reasonable diagnosis, of course, is plasmacytoma.

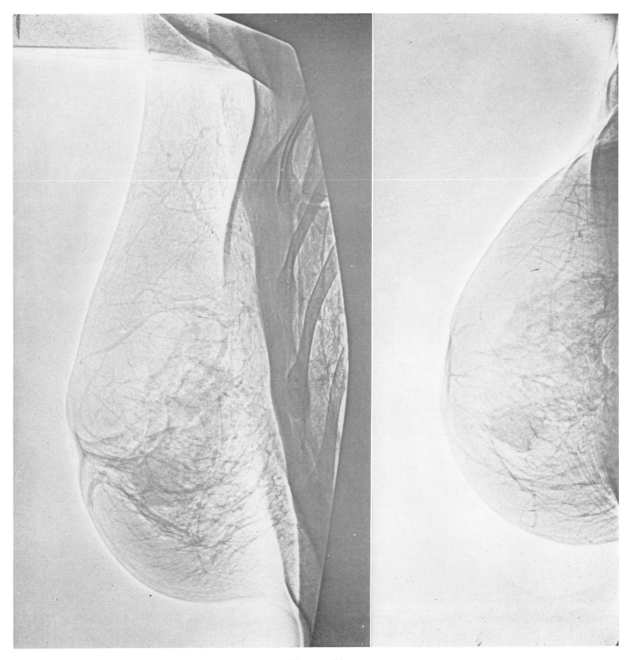

Figure 28.

HISTORY: A sixty-six-year-old, nulliparous woman had a palpable mass in the inner quadrant of the left breast and an indeterminate clinical impression.

RADIOGRAPHIC OBSERVATIONS: The mass in the medial quadrant of the left breast was readily identified (A, B, C). Close inspection of its margin revealed no sharp area of circumscription and the mass faded into the breast parenchyma. There was no pronounced nodularity. There was a suggestion in the lateral projection of some contiguous ducts with the subareolar area, not evidenced, however, on the caudal projection.

A mass in the opposite breast was located in the medial quadrant (C, D, F). It was much smaller, being only 6 mm in size. However, close inspection of it revealed its margin was also somewhat indistinct.

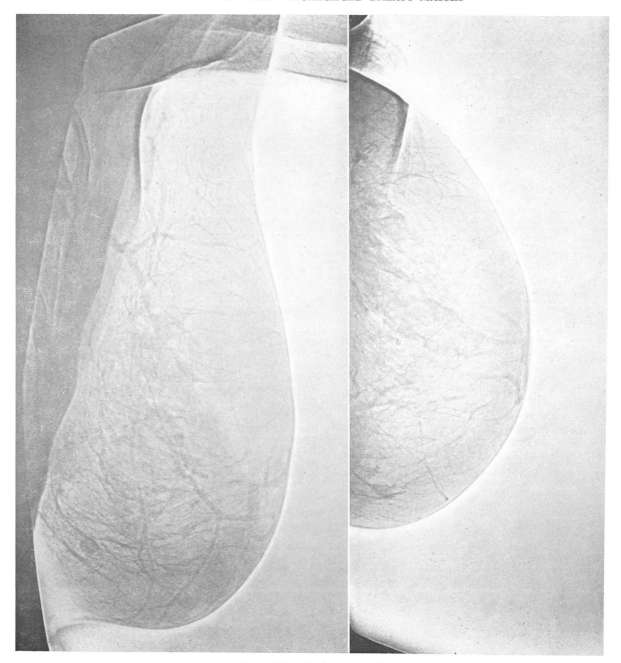

Figure 28 C-D *(Continued)*

IMPRESSION: Bilateral carcinoma suspected.

HISTOPATHOLOGY: Bilateral malignant lymphoma, lymphocytic type.

DISCUSSION: The patient did not have systemic signs of lymphoma. In a few instances of lymphoma which have been observed in the breast, the involvement has been rather diffuse without producing distinct masses. This case is considered very unusual, and the error in diagnosis is considered unavoidable in view of the margins of the masses.

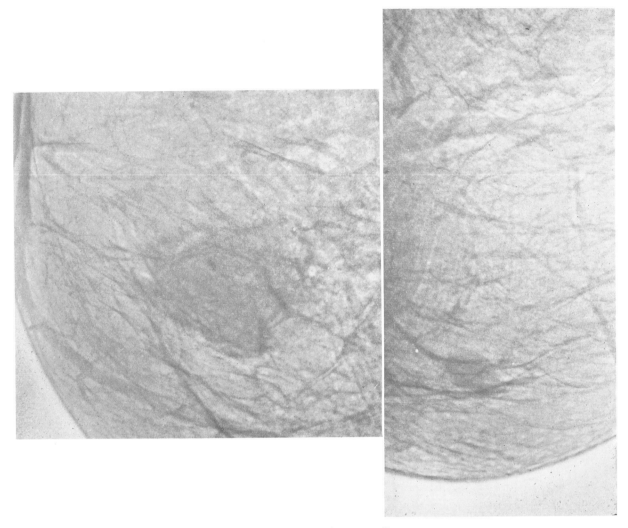

Figure 28 E-F *(Continued)*

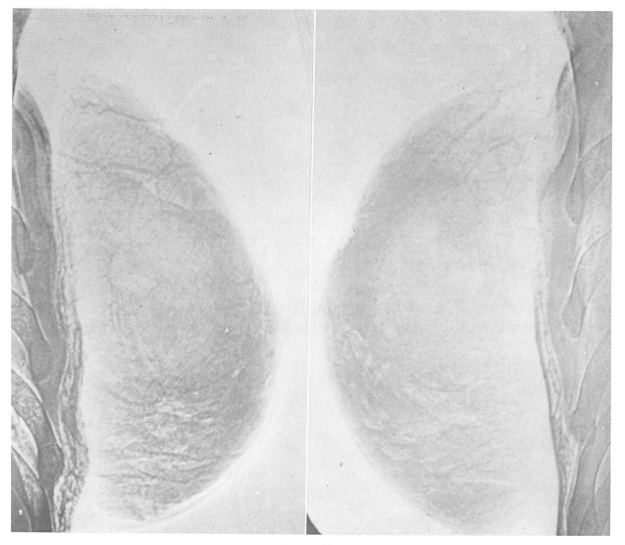

Figure 29.

HISTORY: A twenty-nine-year-old woman discovered masses in the upper axillary quadrants of both breasts. The clinical impression was benign disease.

RADIOGRAPHIC OBSERVATIONS: Figures A and B represent the original examination. The breasts were noted to be involved severely with mammary dysplasia. No evidence of malignancy was seen.

Figure C represents the left breast of the patient three months after biopsy. The very large mass noted on physical examination was observed. The margins of the mass were seen to be sharp and distinct and no clear evidence of carcinoma could be identified.

IMPRESSION: Initial study: benign disease of the breast. Follow-up study: probable hematoma as a result of biopsy.

HISTOPATHOLOGY: Initial study: medullary carcinoma of the breast illustrated in Figure 29A and fibrocystic disease of the opposite breast. Subsequent biopsy of the remaining breast: reticulum cell sarcoma.

Review of the original sections revealed reticulum cell sarcoma on the initial slides rather than medullary carcinoma.

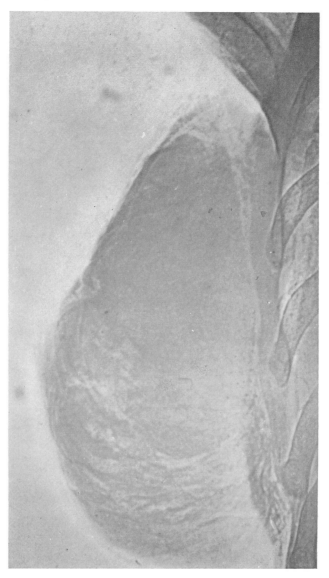

Figure 29 C *(Continued)*

DISCUSSION: It is not possible to arrive at a correct diagnosis of reticulum cell sarcoma on the initial studies of the breast. There are no distinguishing features and the density of the breast parenchyma precludes observation of a mass.

Interpretation of the mass on the second examination of the remaining breast as a hematoma seemed reasonable. The mass arose rather quickly and attained a large size which is not at all unusual for hematoma.

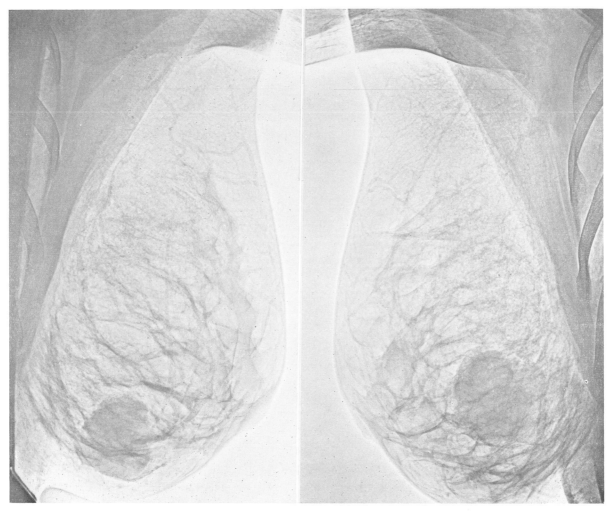

Figure 30.

HISTORY: A thirty-one-year-old, gravida 2 woman who discovered masses in both breasts. She had multiple myeloma.

RADIOGRAPHIC OBSERVATIONS: The sharply circumscribed masses were very evident. There was nothing seen to suggest a malignancy.

IMPRESSION: Bilateral fibroadenomas.

HISTOPATHOLOGY: Bilateral plasmacytomas.

DISCUSSION: Plasmacytomas have an appearance very similar to that of fibroadenomas. In patients who have multiple myeloma, plasmacytomas should be the first impression.

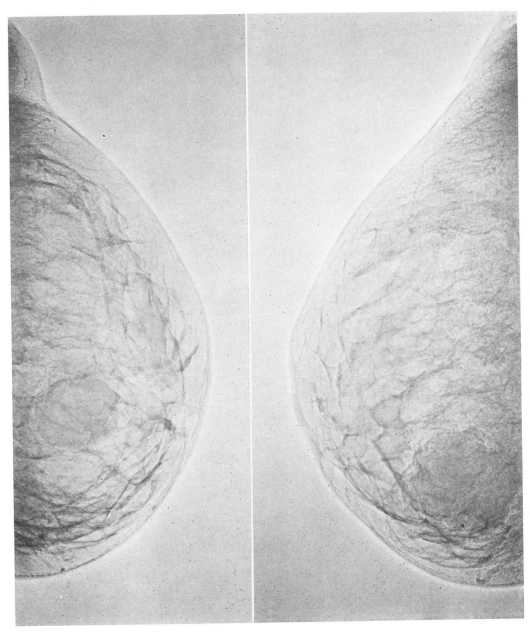

Figure 30 C-D (*Continued*)

Chapter V

Discrete Benign Breast Masses

THE RADIOLOGIST is constantly faced with discrete breast masses of a benign nature. Some benign types are listed below.

1. Intramammary Lymph Node
2. Fibroadenoma
3. Cyst
4. Abscess
5. Papilloma
6. Hematoma
7. Lipoma
8. Galactocele
9. Epidermal Inclusion Cyst
10. Fat Necrosis

Intramammary lymph nodes are probably the most common with fibroadenomas and cysts also having a very high incidence.

The problem is, of course, not to miss the occasional carcinoma which may simulate exactly many of these tumors. Toward that end, all information is used; not only the radiographic appearance of the mass but also the historical features and physical findings.

Often the radiologist will need an interval examination, preferably at three months, and as stated before, the report should be as firm as possible, based on the available information. As always, however, the referring physician must act on the evidence presented by the radiologist and that gained from his own physical examination.

Chapter VI

Intramammary Lymph Nodes

INTRAMAMMARY LYMPH NODES usually do not present problems in diagnosis. They characteristically occur in the upper axillary quadrant of the breast. They are bilateral and are small in size, and they often have a hilar notch. When the hilus is replaced by fat, the lymphoid tissue has a horseshoe configuration around the periphery of the node, and the diagnosis is exceedingly simple.

To be considered normal they should be small, characteristically 5 to 6 millimeters in diameter. Although most often they are single, at times 6 or 8 of them can be identified in both breasts. As a rule, other lymph nodes can be identified both in the axilla and also frequently on the lateral image located near the chest wall. These latter nodes are in the lateral thoracic chain and are extremely difficult to image on the caudal projection, whereas the nodes in the upper axillary quadrant should be imaged on it routinely. (Figs. 31, 32, 33, 34)

They are occasionally involved with metastatic disease, in which case the carcinoma within the breast is usually visible. Typically, when involved with metastases, the node is larger, being a centi-meter or so in size, very oval and solid without fat in the hilus. The notch will usually, but not always, disappear. (Figs. 35, 36)

Care should be exercised in cases of unilateral, especially single, masses. While the most probable etiology of a small, unilateral mass in the upper axillary quadrant is intramammary lymph node, the possibilities of the presence of a very small carcinoma or early node involvement with metastatic neoplastic disease should be entertained. Infrequently, a carcinoma will present in this area as a discrete 3 to 5 millimeter mass. An interval examination after three months should be requested if no biopsy is done. (Fig. 37)

Occasionally the size of the intramammary lymph node can be up to 1½ or 2 centimeters in diameter. They are not always in the upper axillary quadrant either. They may be located anywhere in the breast. In that instance it is impossible to make a correct diagnosis, but the tumors are almost always identified as being benign; usually as either cysts or fibroadenomas. (Fig. 38)

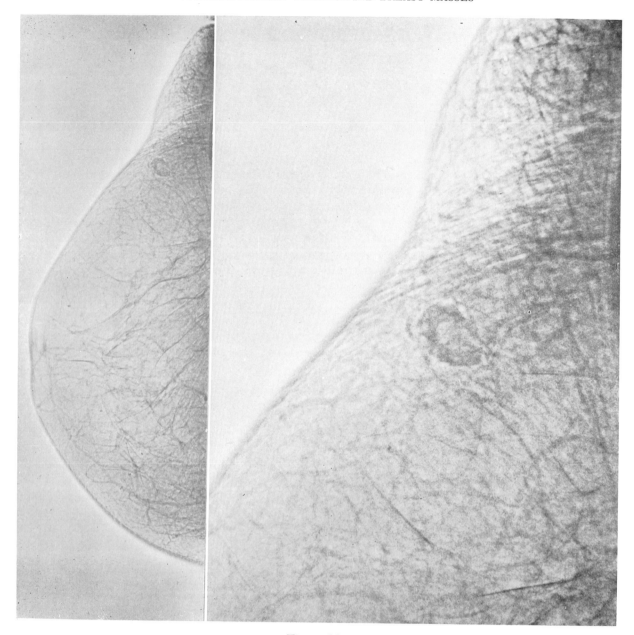

Figure 31.

HISTORY: A fifty-three-year-old, gravida 2 woman complained of pain in the left breast.

RADIOGRAPHIC OBSERVATIONS: The breasts were considered normal. They are composed mainly of fat, but a small mass in the upper axillary quadrant is evident. It has a radiolucent center and a dense periphery.

IMPRESSION: Intramammary lymph node.

HISTOPATHOLOGY: None.

DISCUSSION: Intramammary lymph nodes are very commonly observed in the upper axillary quadrant. Partial replacement by an ingrowth of fat into the hilus leads one to a confident diagnosis.

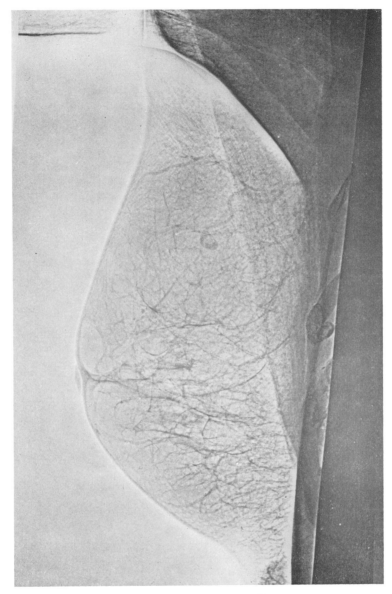

Figure 31 C *(Continued)*

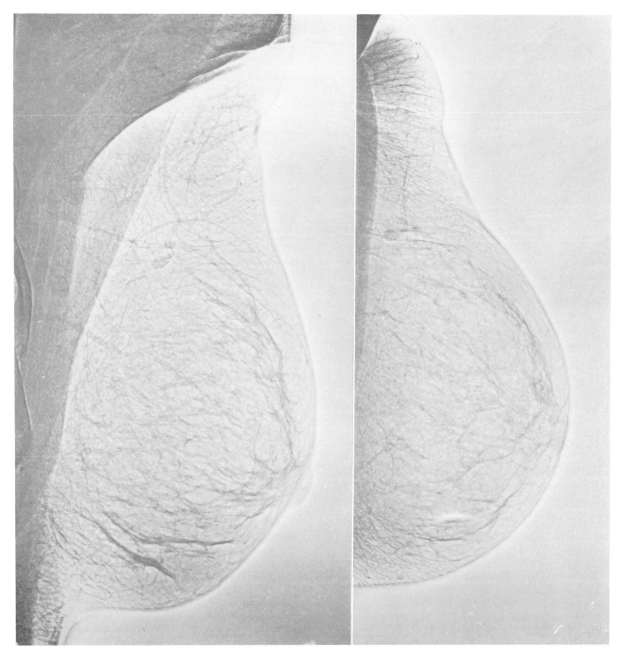

Figure 32.

HISTORY: A fifty-nine-year-old, gravida 2 woman had slight thickening in both breasts and a clinical impression of benign disease.

RADIOGRAPHIC OBSERVATIONS: Both breasts were noted to be composed mainly of fat. Small masses were seen in the upper axillary quadrants of both breasts, two were on the right side.

IMPRESSION: Intramammary lymph nodes.

HISTOPATHOLOGY: None.

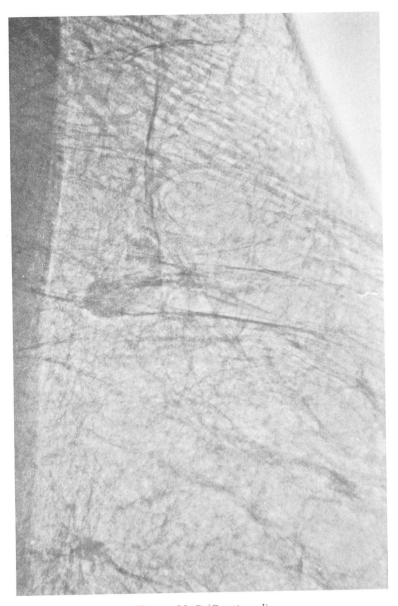

Figure 32 C *(Continued)*

DISCUSSION: Intramammary lymph nodes occur very frequently in this position. Their size and configuration revealed their true nature. The bilaterality is significant. If one small, solid mass were present unilaterally, the need for caution would be greater and follow-up examination should be recommended if no biopsy is performed.

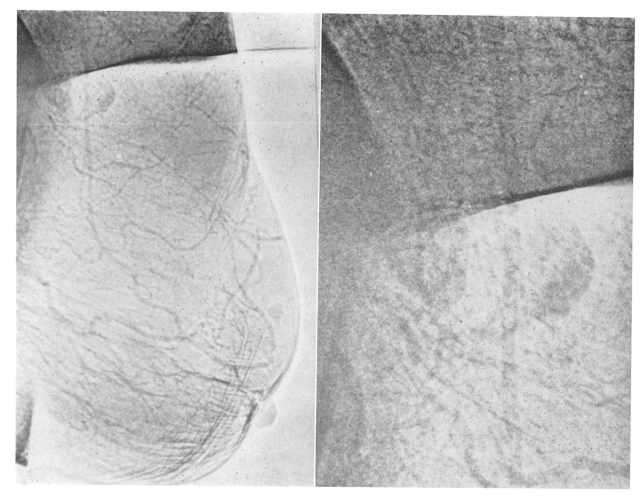

Figure 33.

HISTORY: A sixty-eight-year-old, gravida 6 woman had slight thickening palpable in both breasts and a clinical impression of benign disease. She had a mole near the nipple of the right breast.

RADIOGRAPHIC OBSERVATIONS: The breasts were noted to be composed mainly of fat which placed the patient in a low-risk category for developing a breast cancer. The masses in the upper axillary quadrants had an appearance very characteristic of lymph nodes.

The small mass near the nipple on the right side was observed and, in view of the history and observations by the technologist, it could be placed in the skin.

IMPRESSION: Lymph nodes.

HISTOPATHOLOGY: None.

DISCUSSION: Lymph nodes in elderly women, especially in those who are somewhat obese, tend to be large, sometimes measuring 3 to 4 cms in diameter. There is almost always some degree of replacement by fat, at times to the point where only a rim of lymphoid tissue remains.

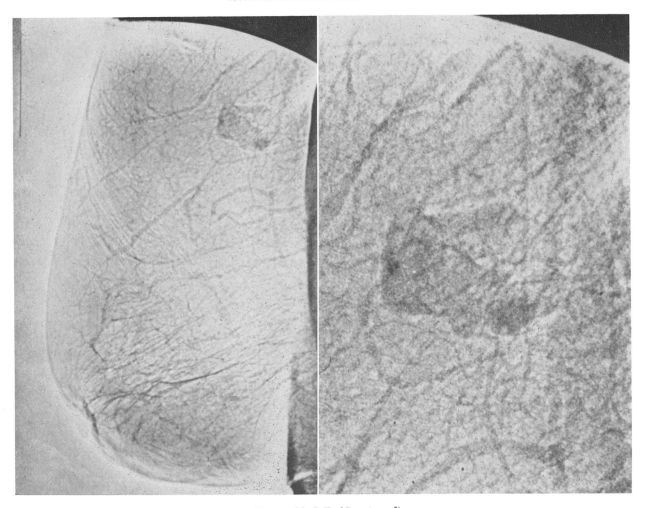

Figure 33 C-D *(Continued)*

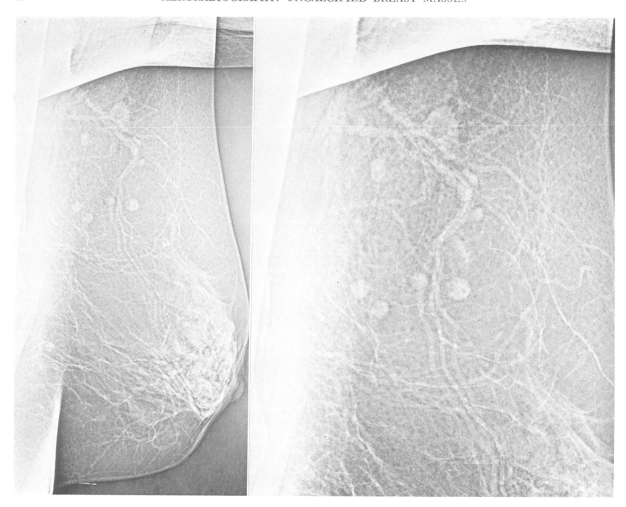

Figure 34.

HISTORY: A seventy-one-year-old, gravida 1 woman had masses palpable in the upper axillary quadrant of the left breast.

RADIOGRAPHIC OBSERVATIONS: Prominent ducts were noted in the subareolar areas of both breasts. The most interesting observation concerned the multiple masses in the upper axillary quadrants. They were bilateral and rather symmetrical. There were similar masses higher into the axilla. All of the masses had sharp margins and in some a notch, representing a hilus, could be seen.

IMPRESSION: Intramammary lymph nodes.

HISTOPATHOLOGY: None.

DISCUSSION: The impression is considered rather straightforward. The location, bilaterality and symmetry of the masses together with other masses being seen higher in the axilla leads one to the logical conclusion that all of the masses represent intramammary lymph nodes. One should, of course, inspect the margin of each mass individually to be certain that one of them does not represent a small carcinoma.

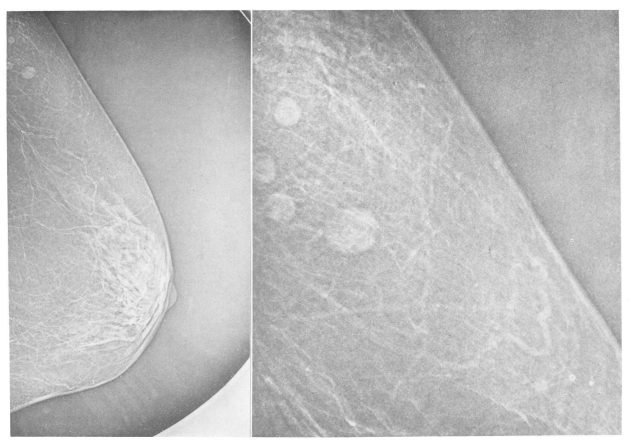

Figure 34 C-D *(Continued)*

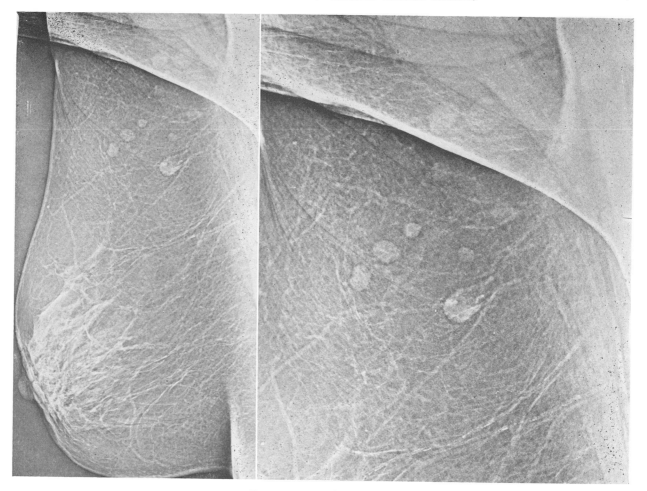

Figure 34 E-F *(Continued)*

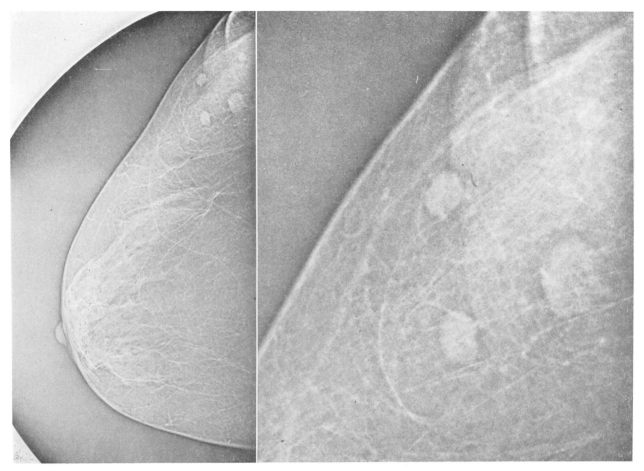

Figure 34 G-H *(Continued)*

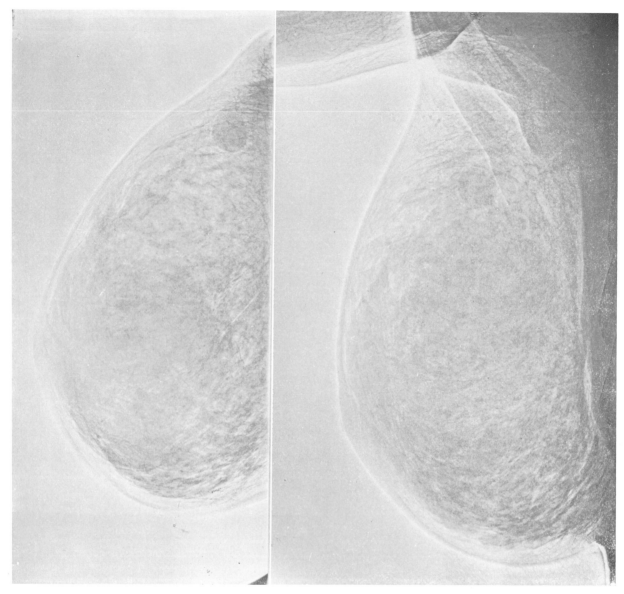

Figure 35.

HISTORY: A thirty-nine-year-old, gravida 2 woman discovered a lump in her left breast. The clinical impression was indeterminate.

RADIOGRAPHIC OBSERVATIONS: There were two abnormalites to be considered; the most obvious was the mass identified in the upper axillary quadrant. It was sharply circumscribed and in the usual location for an intramammary lymph node. It was larger than the normal intramammary lymph node.

The second observation was the mass-like density in the central portion of the breast, seen best on the caudal projection. This area of asymmetry was identified by comparison with the opposite breast. In addition, both breasts were involved severely with a prominent duct pattern.

IMPRESSION: Large carcinoma, central portion of the breast with the possibility of metastases to an intramammary lymph node.

HISTOPATHOLOGY: Carcinoma of the breast (tubular and scirrhous) and metastases to one lymph node.

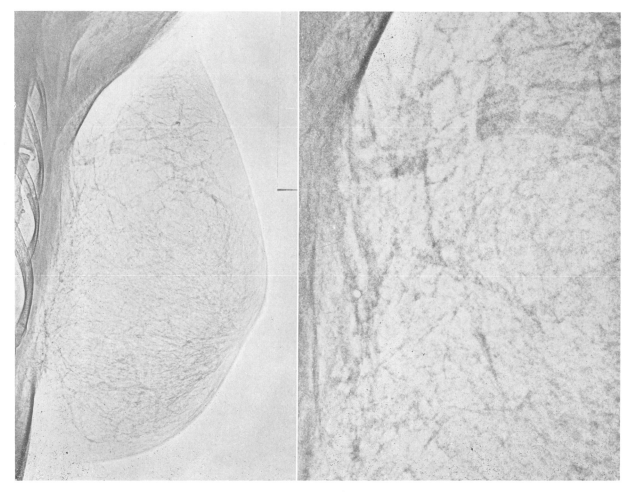

Figure 37.

HISTORY: A sixty-three-year-old, gravida 2 woman discovered an area of thickness in the axillary portion of her right breast. The physical examination was not remarkable at that time, but six months later a definite mass was palpable in the upper axillary quadrant. The clinical impression was carcinoma.

RADIOGRAPHIC OBSERVATIONS: On the first study the only abnormality that was noted was the small mass readily visible in the upper portion of the breast. It was noted to be sharply circumscribed and no radiographic features of carcinoma could be identified (A).

On the study made six months later, a definite irregular mass was observed that had replaced the small mass. In addition, lymph nodes became visible in the axilla (B).

IMPRESSION: The first study resulted in the mass being interpreted as an intramammary lymph node. On the second study a carcinoma was obvious with probable metastases to the axillary lymph nodes.

HISTOPATHOLOGY: Carcinoma with metastases to six lymph nodes.

DISCUSSION: On the first examination diagnosis is exceedingly difficult. The mass has the usual appearance of an intramammary lymph node being sharply circumscribed and in the right location. No mass was seen in the opposite breast, however. In retrospect, one might have requested a reexamination after an interval of three to four months or been more cognizant of the unilaterality and roundness of the mass and above all the palpable abnormality. It is an error which is difficult to avoid.

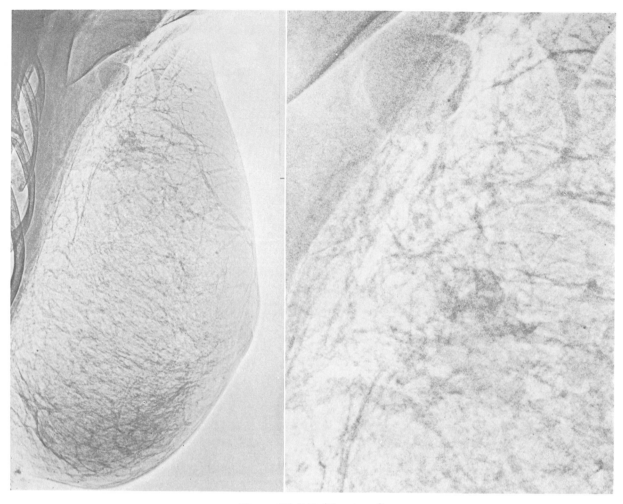

Figure 37 C-D *(Continued)*

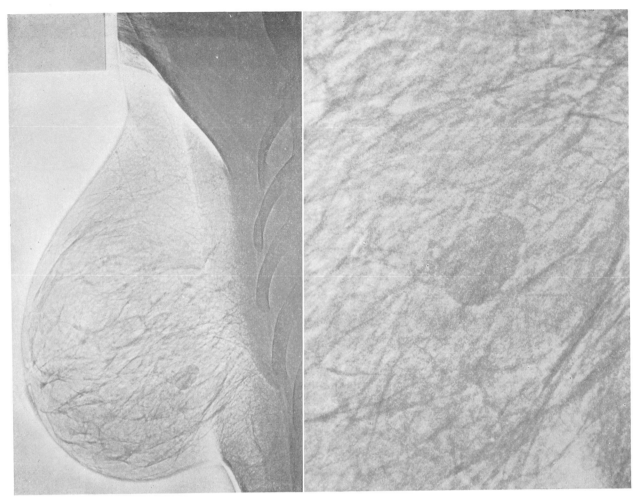

Figure 38.

HISTORY: A twenty-year-old, gravida 1 woman discovered a mass in her left breast. The clinical impression was benign disease.

RADIOGRAPHIC OBSERVATIONS: The rather sharply circumscribed tumor in the axillary quadrant of the left breast was readily observed. The breast itself is noted to be normal apart from the tumor. Because of the age of the patient and the appearance of the mass, it was believed rather firmly to represent a fibroadenoma.

IMPRESSION: Fibroadenoma.

HISTOPATHOLOGY: Heterotopic lymph node.

DISCUSSION: This is an unusual location for an intramammary lymph node. Characteristically they are in the upper axillary quadrant. There is no way to avoid an error such as this. The intramammary lymph node is an ovoid tumor. In a young woman whose breast is otherwise normal, a mass like this would be diagnosed benign, probably a fibroadenoma.

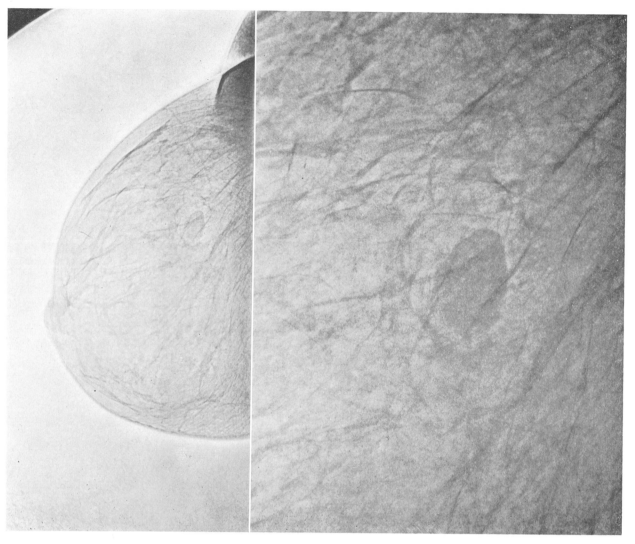

Figure 38 C-D *(Continued)*

Chapter VII

Fibroadenomas

THE TYPICAL CASE OF fibroadenoma will have the following features. The woman is usually young, under the age of thirty-five and often significantly younger, even in her teens. The physical findings are those of a smooth mass which is firm and freely movable. It can be located anywhere in the breast. Multiple fibroadenomas occur in about 35 percent of cases. Bilateral fibroadenomas are similarly common.

Radiographically the mass is readily discernible, except in the occasional case when the breast is extremely dense and there is not sufficient fat to afford the necessary contrast. The tumor is typically lobulated and sharply defined. There may or may not be a radiolucent halo. (The halo is not considered pathognomic of fibroadenoma as it occurs in many other tumors, especially cysts and, rarely, in medullary carcinomas.) More often than not, all of the margins will not be seen because the mass is overshadowed by other structures in the breast. One should, however, diagnose what is most probable. Failing to see a portion of the wall when there is no real evidence of malignancy should not deter one from a firm impression of fibroadenoma if the segments of the wall that are seen are extremely sharp and typical for the tumor. (Figs. 39, 40, 41, 42, 43, 44, 45)

Fibroadenomas can be seen in any age group, although there are several characteristic situations in which they are frequently observed; notably, the giant fibroadenoma of the teenager and those that are associated with pregnancy or lactation. Neither of these usually pose any problems in diagnosis. (Figs. 46, 47)

The lactating adenoma is, of course, associated with lactation. Its appearance is not unlike that of other fibroadenomas. Characteristically, these are sharply circumscribed tumors with a gently lobular margin. Often a halo of compressed fat can be seen. They rarely contain calcifications. Lactating adenomas are so characteristic that it is extremely unusual to overcall them as malignant tumors. (Figs. 48, 49)

Giant fibroadenomas in the young are notable for their very large size when first observed. It is not uncommon to see them in girls at the age of 15 or 16, and often the breast containing the fibroadenoma is two to three times larger than the opposite normal one. Here, again, their appearance is consistent, being sharply circumscribed, uncalcified and usually displacing adjacent breast tissue. At times they are very lobulated, simulating somewhat the marked lobularity seen in cystosarcoma phylloides. Calcifications have not been observed except in one 25-year-old woman who had had the tumor for eight years. (Fig. 50)

Lipofibroadenomas and adenolipomas have perfectly characteristic radiographic features and present absolutely no problem in diagnosis. They have not been observed to calcify. The lipofibroadenoma is a nonhomogeneous mass which has densities corresponding to fat and epithelial and connective tissue. It is sharply limited, and one can usually discern a faint, thin capsule. They are not common tumors, only thirty cases having been observed in 50,000 examinations at Hutzel Hospital.

Adenolipomas are extremely rare but, when seen, have an appearance which cannot be confused with carcinoma. They are sharply limited, nonhomogeneous tumors containing primarily fat with added epithelial and connective tissue densities. (Fig. 51)

There are many fibroadenomas, however, which resemble carcinoma rather closely, and often it is impossible to come to a correct diagnosis. Some of them will have distinctly nodular margins, and when confronted with such a tumor, especially if the woman is in the cancer-prone age group, one must suspect a medullary carcinoma. (Figs. 52, 53)

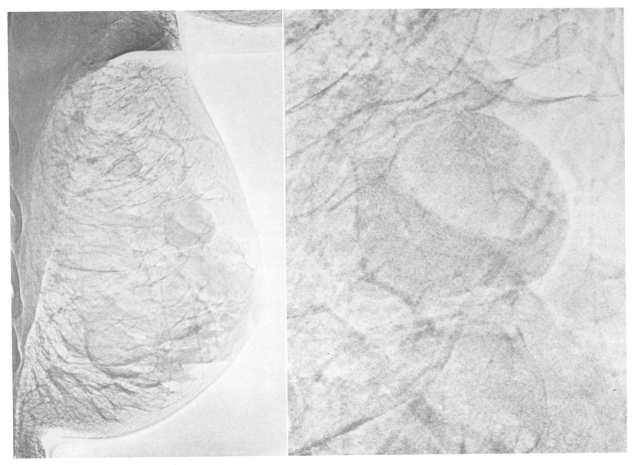

Figure 39.

HISTORY: A thirty-one-year-old, gravida 4 woman discovered a mass in her right breast. The clinical impression was benign disease.

RADIOGRAPHIC OBSERVATIONS: The breasts were noted to be involved with minor degrees of mammary dysplasia. The mass in the upper axillary quadrant on the right was readily visible. Most of its margins could be seen when one considered both projections and in all observed segments it was noted to be extremely sharp and well defined. Failure to observe the mass in its entirety was believed due to overshadowing structures within the breast. Note also that there was a smaller mass in the subareolar area which was somewhat lobulated.

IMPRESSION: Two fibroadenomas.

HISTOPATHOLOGY: Fibroadenomas.

DISCUSSION: The multiplicity of the masses, their lobulation and sharp circumscription should lead one into the correct impression of fibroadenoma especially in view of the history. The youth and multiparity of the woman make carcinoma unlikely.

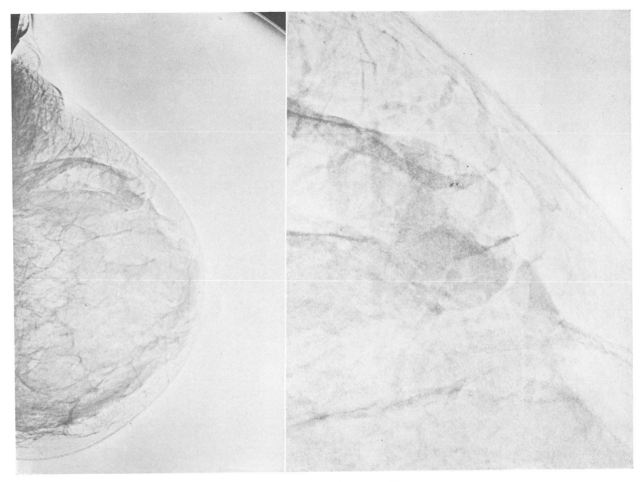

Figure 39 C-D *(Continued)*

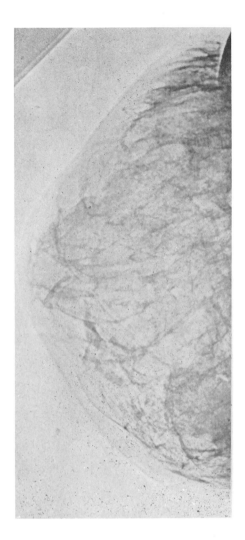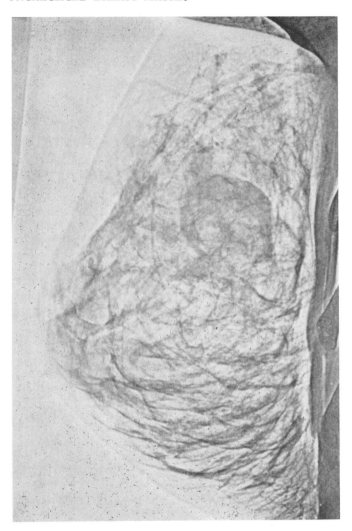

Figure 40.

HISTORY: A nineteen-year-old, gravida 2 woman had a mass palpable in the left breast.

RADIOGRAPHIC OBSERVATIONS: The breasts were considered to be involved with very minor degrees of mammary dysplasia. The main observation concerned the mass which appeared to be lobulated and had very sharp margins.

IMPRESSION: Fibroadenoma.

HISTOPATHOLOGY: Fibroadenoma.

DISCUSSION: The lobulation and sharp circumscription of this tumor in a young woman should lead to a very firm diagnosis of fibroadenoma.

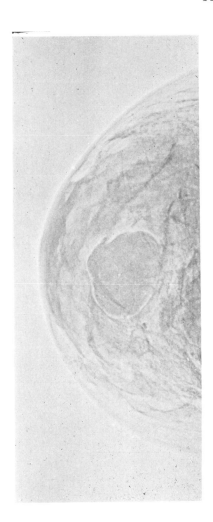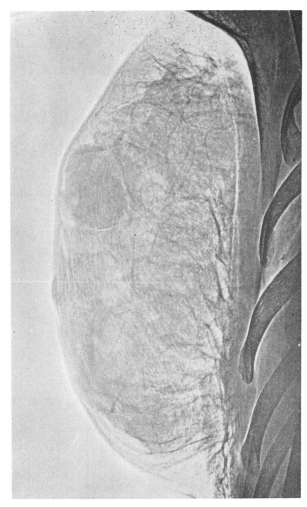

Figure 41.

HISTORY: A nineteen-year-old, gravida 1 woman discovered a mass in her left breast. The physical examination revealed the tumor to be readily palpable and the impression was that of benign disease.

RADIOGRAPHIC OBSERVATIONS: The overall appearance of the breast, being very dense, was that of severe mammary dysplasia. This is not an unusual observation in a young woman. The tumor could be readily identified. It was noted to have a sharp margin with a radiolucent halo and it bulged the skin but did not produce any change in the skin.

IMPRESSION: Fibroadenoma.

HISTOPATHOLOGY: Fibroadenoma.

DISCUSSION: A discrete tumor in a nineteen-year-old woman almost always represents a fibroadenoma. The appearance of the tumor, of course, is very characteristic.

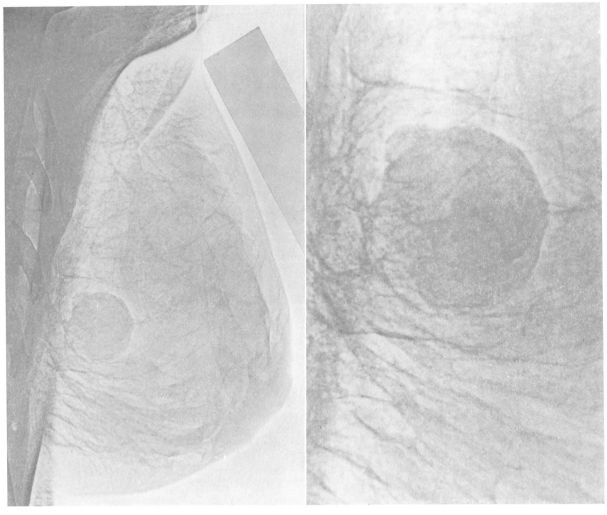

Figure 42.

HISTORY: A twenty-six-year-old, gravida 1 woman had biopsies of both breasts six years before the study. She now complains of a lump in the right breast in the lateral aspect.

RADIOGRAPHIC OBSERVATIONS: The mass, which contained no calcifications, was located rather deeply near the chest wall. It was readily identified. It was noted to have a lobulated appearance with a very sharp and distinct margin visible in two projections.

IMPRESSION: Fibroadenoma.

HISTOPATHOLOGY: Fibroadenoma.

DISCUSSION: The lobulated appearance of the margin of the mass and the age of the patient lead one into the correct radiographic impression of fibroadenoma.

Located above and slightly anterior to the mass are a few relatively large calcifications which are the remnants of another fibroadenoma which had undergone degeneration.

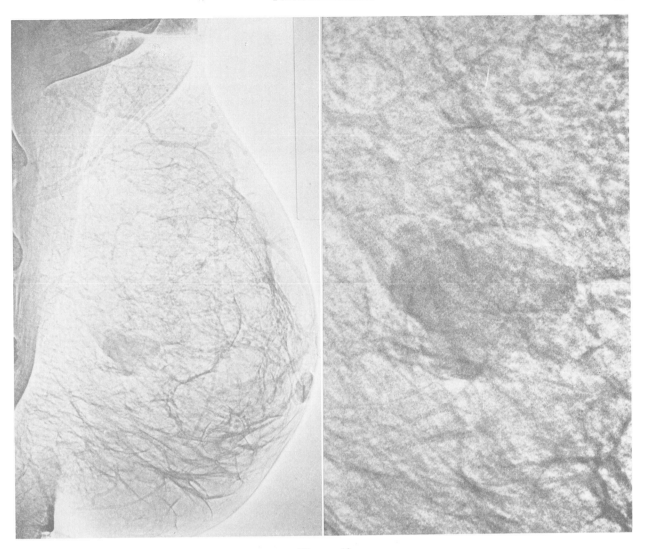

Figure 43.

HISTORY: A twenty-five-year-old, gravida 2 woman had a biopsy of the right breast eight months before this examination and now has a mass palpable in the right breast.

RADIOGRAPHIC OBSERVATIONS: Both breasts were noted to be composed mainly of fat. A mass in the axillary portion of the right breast was readily identified. It seemed to be somewhat lobulated with very indistinct medial and anterior margins and some anterior tapering.

IMPRESSION: Fibroadenoma with an outside possibility of carcinoma. It was recommended if the mass was not excised, the patient should be followed very carefully.

HISTOPATHOLOGY: Fibroadenoma.

DISCUSSION: Lobulated masses in young women are almost always fibroadenomas. However, when a considerable portion of the margin of the mass, especially in a fatty breast, is indistinct, one must consider that it might represent a carcinoma.

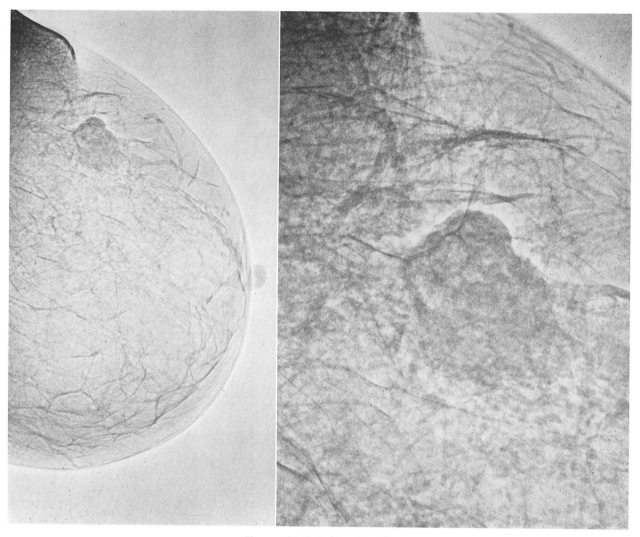

Figure 43 C-D *(Continued)*

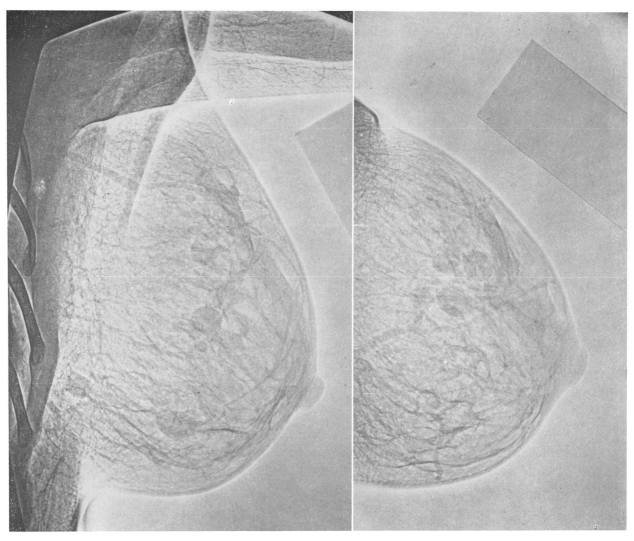

Figure 44.

HISTORY: A twenty-one-year-old, gravida 1 woman discovered a mass in the axillary quadrant of the left breast.

RADIOGRAPHIC OBSERVATIONS: Multiple, sharply circumscribed masses were readily identified within both breasts. None contained calcifications. The general appearance of the breast was that of an essentially normal parenchyma.

IMPRESSION: Multiple fibroadenomas.

HISTOPATHOLOGY: Fibroadenomas.

DISCUSSION: The soft tissue masses are sharply circumscribed. Some of these masses tend to be lobular. When they are multiple and bilateral in young women, they are almost always fibroadenomas.

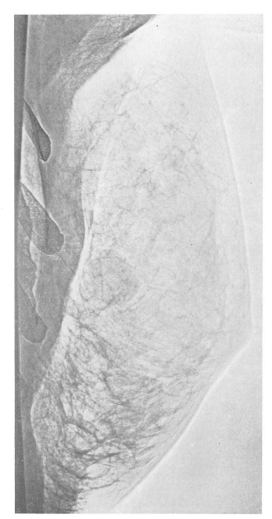
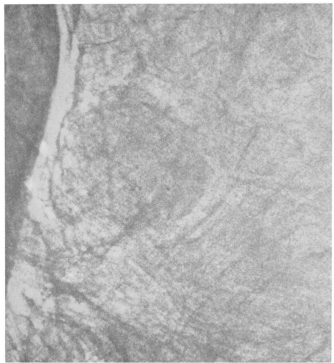

Figure 45.

HISTORY: A twenty-nine-year-old, nulliparous woman complained of a clear discharge from both breasts.

RADIOGRAPHIC OBSERVATIONS: The breasts were seen to be involved with moderate amounts of mammary dysplasia. The mass in the axillary half of the right breast was readily identified. The mass was noted to be lobular and at least 50 percent of its margin could be identified as benign. It was very sharp in the caudal projection.

IMPRESSION: Fibroadenoma.

HISTOPATHOLOGY: Fibroadenoma.

DISCUSSION: Lobulated tumors in young women are almost always fibroadenomas. The failure to see all of the margin of the mass can be attributed to coexistent mammary dysplasia which obscures portions of the margin. One can base the weight of his opinion on the sharpness of the margin that is free from overlying or underlying dysplasia.

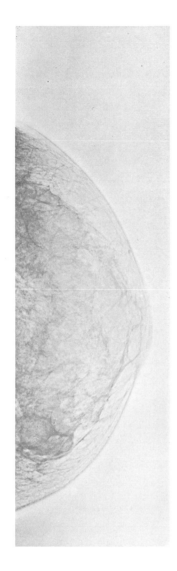

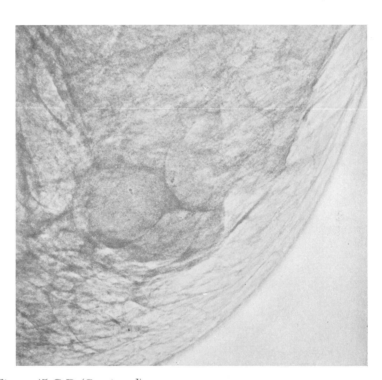

Figure 45 C-D *(Continued)*

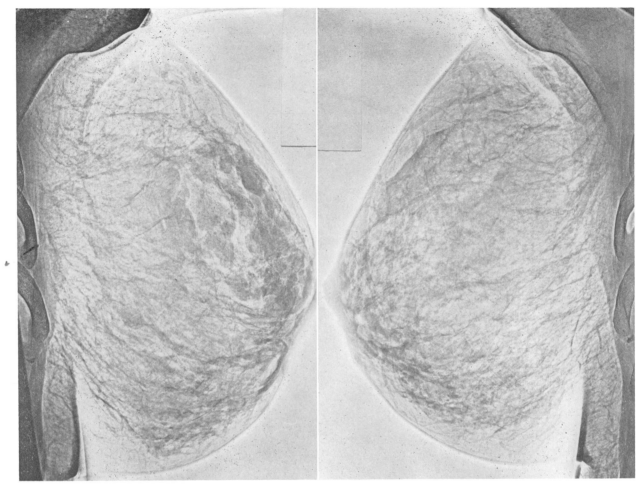

Figure 46.

HISTORY: A thirty-five-year-old, gravida 2 woman had palpated a mass in the upper portion of the right breast. The clinical impression was that of benign disease.

RADIOGRAPHIC OBSERVATIONS: The general condition of the breast was regarded as being involved with minor degrees of mammary dyplasia. The nonhomogeneous, somewhat cauliflower-appearing mass beginning in the subareolar area and extending superiorly and posteriorly over an area of about 5 cm was noted to have a very thin capsule-like structure surrounding it.

IMPRESSION: Lipofibroadenoma, right breast.

HISTOPATHOLOGY: Lipofibroadenoma.

DISCUSSION: Lipofibroadenomas constitute probably less than 1 percent of all fibroadenomas. One can usually identify a thin, capsule-like structure around at least portions of the tumor.

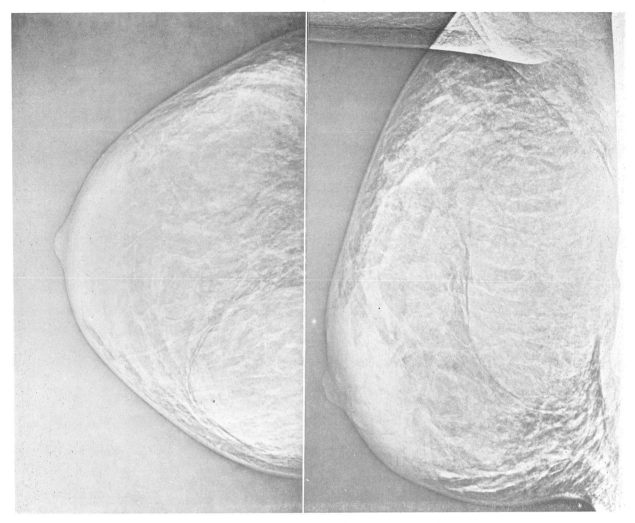

Figure 47.

HISTORY: An eighteen-year-old, nulliparous woman, five months pregnant, discovered a large mass in her left breast.

RADIOGRAPHIC OBSERVATIONS: The changes of pregnancy were noted evidenced by the general increase in density to the parenchyma of the breast. A large mass which is sharply circumscribed was seen. No evidence of carcinoma was discovered.

IMPRESSION: Lactating adenoma.

HISTOPATHOLOGY: Lactating adenoma.

DISCUSSION: This type of tumor is exceedingly common in pregnant women and those who are lactating. A confident impression of benignancy can be made on the basis of the very sharp margin, history and physical findings.

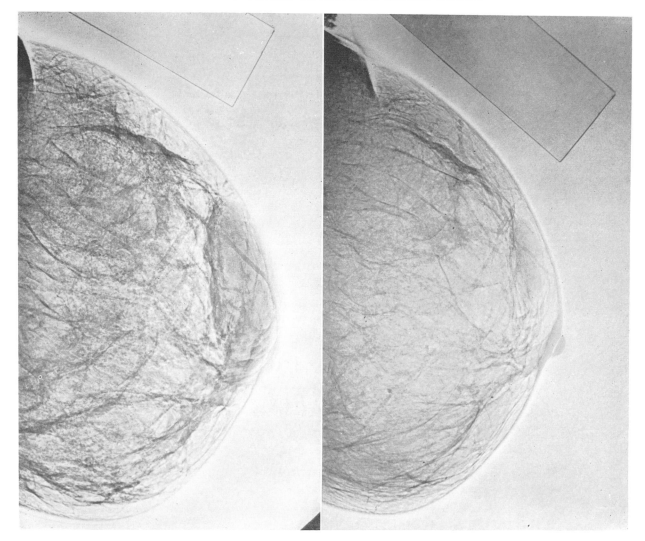

Figure 48.

HISTORY: A thirty-two-year-old, gravida 3 woman, four weeks postpartum, discovered a mass in the right breast.

RADIOGRAPHIC OBSERVATIONS: (A) A superficially-placed subareolar tumor was readily visible. Also present were changes in the breast from pregnancy with prominent vascularity and general increase in density to the parenchyma. The posterior margin of the mass was not perfectly sharp and smooth. However, all things considered, the tumor was judged to be benign.

(B) The breast had reverted to its normal resting state, being composed mainly of fat. The tumor was barely visible, being only one fourth of its original size.

IMPRESSION: Lactating adenoma.

HISTOPATHOLOGY: None.

DISCUSSION: Lactating adenomas are very common in the postpartum woman. Usually they present as rather sharply circumscribed masses, such as this case. These tumors usually regress with the cessation of pregnancy and lactation.

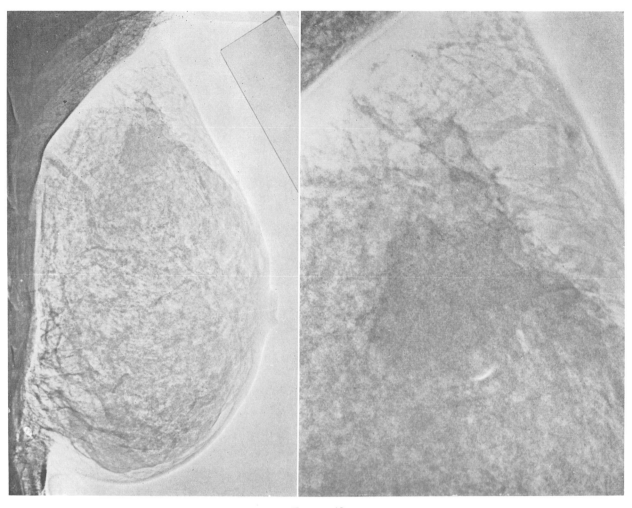

Figure 49.

HISTORY: A twenty-four-year-old, gravida 1 woman palpated a mass in the upper outer quadrant of the right breast. She is two months postpartum.

RADIOGRAPHIC OBSERVATIONS: The general increase in density of the parenchyma is very consistent with lactation. The 2 cm mass was readily identified and noted to have an extremely irregular margin, being in some areas very nodular and in others somewhat spiculated.

IMPRESSION: Carcinoma.

HISTOPATHOLOGY: Lactating adenoma.

DISCUSSION: This is a very unusual case. Lactating adenomas generally are observed as very sharply circumscribed, lobulated tumors. This case was interpreted rather strongly for carcinoma and there is no explanation for a lactating adenoma presented in such a different fashion.

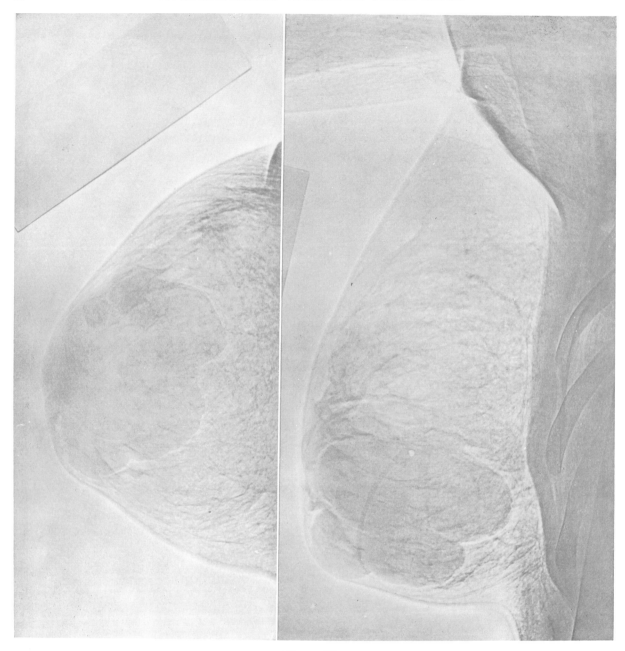

Figure 50.

HISTORY: A fifteen-year-old, nulliparous girl discovered a mass in the lower portion of the left breast. The clinical impression was benign disease.

RADIOGRAPHIC OBSERVATIONS: The breasts are unusual for a fifteen-year-old in that they are composed mainly of fat with very little dysplasia. A multilobulated mass in the subareolar area and lower quadrant which bulged the skin but did not change the skin was observed. No calcifications were seen.

IMPRESSION: Fibroadenoma.

HISTOPATHOLOGY: Fibroadenoma.

DISCUSSION: Marked multilobularity, especially in a fifteen-year-old girl, is an almost certain indicator of fibroadenoma. Exceptions are very rare.

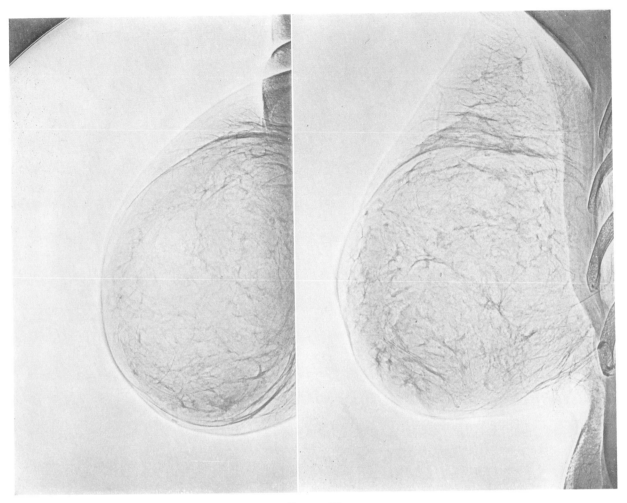

Figure 51.

HISTORY: A fifty-year-old, nulliparous woman has noted for a long time that the left breast was larger than the right. She also had slight pain.

RADIOGRAPHIC OBSERVATIONS: The chief observation made was the very faint capsule evidenced by a sharp line superiorly and inferiorly and with a very slight relative radiolucency with areas of density within it.

IMPRESSION: Adenolipoma.

HISTOPATHOLOGY: Adenolipoma.

DISCUSSION: The case represents a very large adenolipoma, which is unusual. In addition to being composed merely of fat; there are added epithelial or connective tissue densities within it.

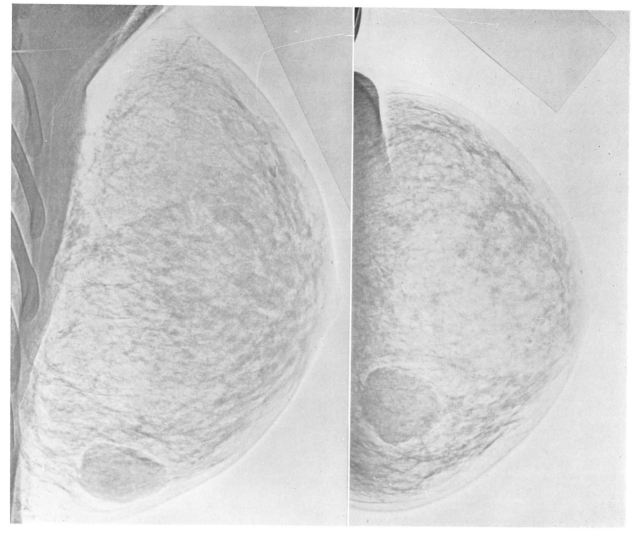

Figure 52.

HISTORY: A twenty-four-year-old, nulliparous woman discovered a lump in the left breast.

RADIOGRAPHIC OBSERVATIONS: Both breasts were noted to be involved with what appeared to be a prominent duct pattern. This was considered significant. The mass was apparent and its margin appeared very nodular in areas.

IMPRESSION: Possible medullary carcinoma but more likely a fibroadenoma.

HISTOPATHOLOGY: Fibroadenoma.

DISCUSSION: Medullary carcinomas, as well as all other carcinomas, are infrequently observed in the very young woman. Fibroadenomas are most commonly found in this age group. Although the most likely diagnosis was fibroadenoma, because of the nodular margin of the mass, excision, or as a second choice, reexamination, was recommended.

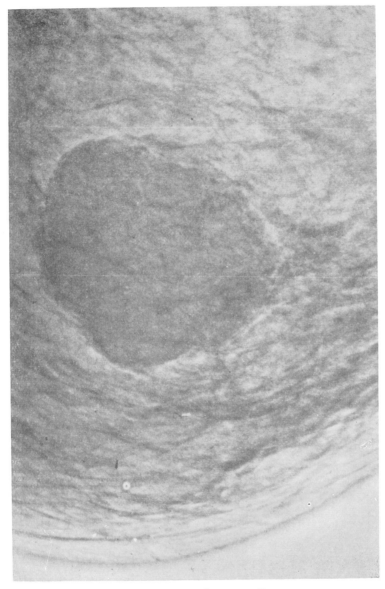

Figure 52 C *(Continued)*

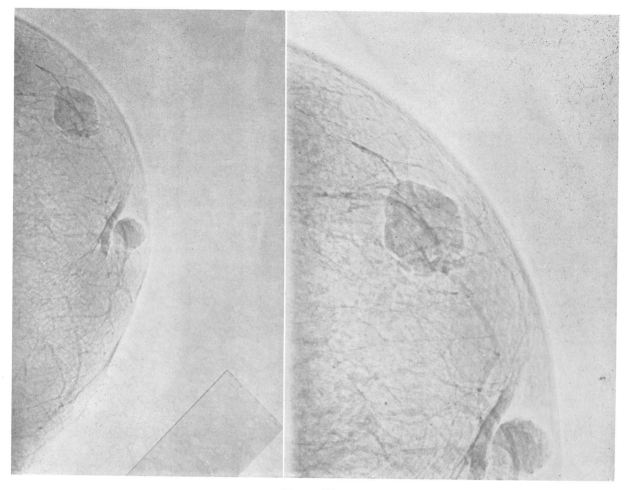

Figure 53.

HISTORY: A forty-nine-year-old, nulliparous woman had a right mastectomy nineteen years before this study. She discovered a mass in the remaining breast.

RADIOGRAPHIC OBSERVATIONS: The breast was composed almost completely of fat so the patient was at low-risk for developing a second breast cancer. The mass, however, was noted to be somewhat nodular in areas and was regarded with suspicion.

IMPRESSION: Suspicion for medullary carcinoma.

HISTOPATHOLOGY: Fibroadenoma.

DISCUSSION: It is difficult to avoid an error such as this. Most likely, the mass represents a benign tumor. Although the breast is composed mainly of fat which reduces the risk of carcinoma, the patient's age and history of breast cancer make aspiration or excision the necessary mode of treatment.

Chapter VIII

Cysts

CYSTS, LIKE FIBROADENOMAS, do not usually present great problems in diagnosis, although certainly a significant number will be suspected of representing a medullary carcinoma or some other form of circumscribed neoplasm. Rarely, some will even lead the observer to a firm diagnosis of carcinoma. Cysts tend to involve an older age group than do fibroadenomas and, for that reason alone, are more suspect of being carcinomas.

The history is very important, as are serial studies of the breast. Typically, the patient discovers a tumor in her breast which "was not there a short time ago." This is very possibly an accurate observation but, of course, in itself it is not reliable. Of some importance is the fact that by the time she sees her physician and obtains an appointment for a mammographic examination, often she will state, and again quite accurately, that the cyst has disappeared. This rapid fluctuation in size and number of cysts is characteristic and makes serial examinations extremely important and helpful in the care of the patient. Cysts often will be tender to palpation, freely movable and multiple. The physical findings are not those of the usual carcinoma.

Radiographically one can be confident in a large number of these cases. When a round or very oval mass with an exceedingly sharp margin is observed, especially with the historical features of rapid onset and pain, the interpretation should be confident and direct. (Figs. 54, 55, 56, 57, 58)

Very often not all of the wall of the mass can be seen due to overlapping structures (as in fibroadenoma). Here again, failing to see all of the margin, but also failing to see definitive evidence of malignancy, should lead one to the more probable diagnosis of cyst rather than carcinoma. (Figs. 60, 61, 62, 63, 64, 65, 66, 67)

Cysts are often multiple and bilateral, and this too can be used in decision making. Keep in mind, however, that each mass must be considered individually with its margin closely inspected for spiculation or nodulation, calcifications, and all of the other signs of breast carcinoma. (Fig. 68)

A rapid change (less than 3 months) in a sharply contoured mass is characteristic for cysts rather than solid tumors. It is not unusual to see a 25 percent increase or decrease in size. The configuration and sharpness of the border remain the same. In evaluating any change in the size of a mass, however, care must be taken that the radiographic geometry is kept constant. For example, the object-plate (object-film) distance and degree of compression are extremely important.

It is fortunate that cysts change rapidly as to size, number and bilaterality. It is not uncommon to see a patient initially with a discrete, uncalcified breast mass and to find three months later that the cyst has vanished completely, has increased 50 percent in size, or very often that others have appeared in the same or the opposite breast. It is in the instance of cysts that repeat examinations are the most valuable and a three-month interval is reasonable for this. (Figs. 69, 70, 71)

Unlike a cyst, a circumscribed carcinoma, if it is changing, is more likely to do so in regards to its contour, rather than its size in a short period of time. Longer periods of time, six months or more, may demonstrate clearly a doubling of size of a circumscribed carcinoma. Usually, however, in addition to the increase in size, other signs of carcinoma become much more prominent such as irregular contour, the occurrence of calcifications, edema, etc.

It is important to realize that the rapidly growing carcinoma is one which is characterized by only a slight increase in parenchymal density and not as a discrete mass. This type of carcinoma can easily double or triple in size within six months.

Fibroadenomas change very slowly. Usually when first seen they are as large as one will observe them with a notable exception of the influ-

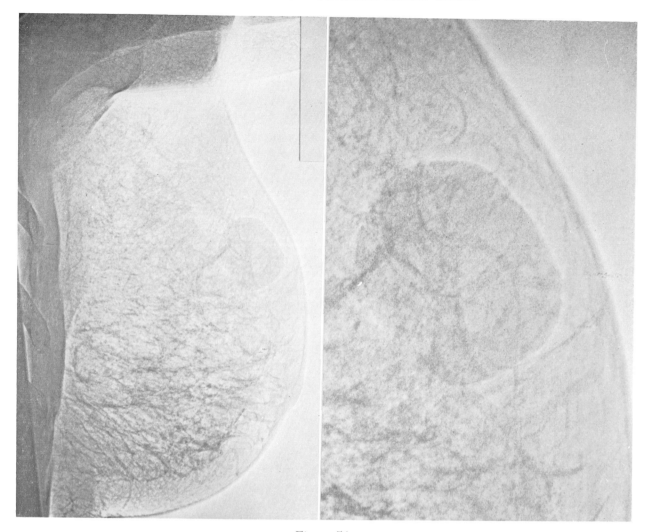

Figure 54.

HISTORY: A thirty-nine-year-old, gravida 2 woman had a mass palpable in the upper portion of the right breast and a clinical impression of benign disease.

RADIOGRAPHIC OBSERVATIONS: The very sharply limited mass was thought to represent a benign tumor mainly on the basis of its extremely smooth margin.

IMPRESSION: Cyst, right breast.

HISTOPATHOLOGY: Cyst.

DISCUSSION: A very sharply outlined ovoid mass in a thirty-nine-year-old woman is most likely a cyst. On a percentage basis, a second choice would be a fibroadenoma. Its superficial location speaks more for a benign tumor than malignancy.

This is the type of mass in which aspiration as a method of diagnosis and treatment is very helpful. It is palpable, superficially placed and aspirating the cyst's contents should be very easy.

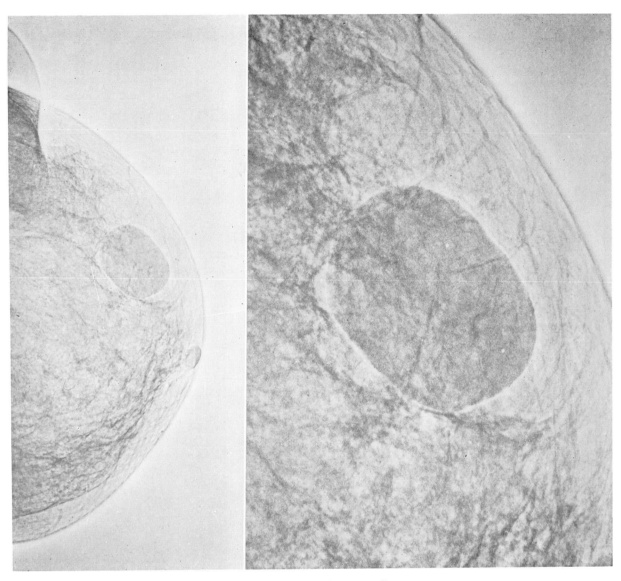

Figure 54 C-D *(Continued)*

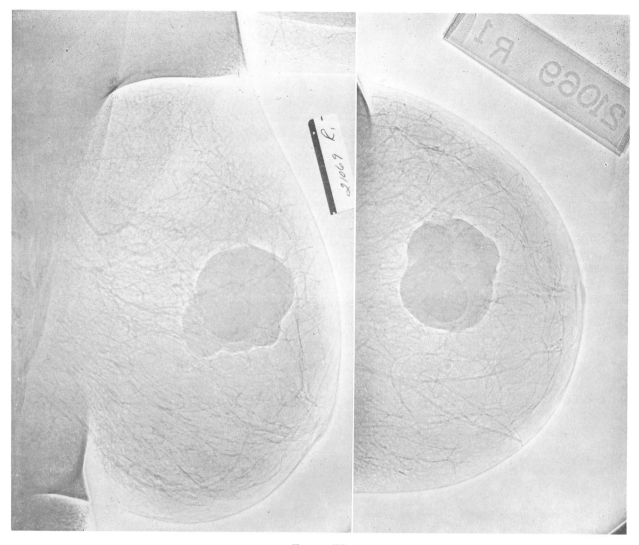

Figure 55.

HISTORY: A fifty-eight-year-old, gravida 4 woman had a mass palpable in the right breast of only four weeks' duration.

RADIOGRAPHIC OBSERVATIONS: The breasts were composed largely of fat with the exception of a mass in the right breast. The mass was noted to be multilobulated. The margins of the mass were seen to be sharp and distinct.

IMPRESSION: Cyst with an outside possibility of medullary carcinoma. Aspiration or excision was recommended. If neither aspiration or excision were performed, careful follow-up examinations were strongly recommended.

HISTOPATHOLOGY: Cyst.

DISCUSSION: The woman was a good observer who routinely examined her breasts. The very short history of only four weeks and sudden appearance would speak for a cyst rather than a carcinoma. It should be recognized, however, that some medullary carcinomas can have an appearance identical to this.

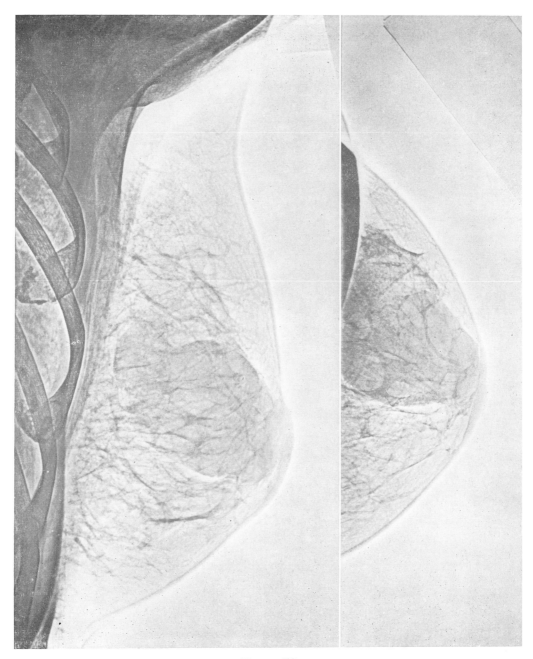

Figure 56.

HISTORY: A forty-one-year-old woman had masses palpable in both breasts, but the changes were more severe on the right. The clinical impression was benign disease.

RADIOGRAPHIC OBSERVATIONS: There were masses in both breasts all of which appeared to have sharp margins to them.

The mass on the right was considered very sharply limited. One can identify most of the borders quite well and there was no irregularity or nodularity.

IMPRESSION: Cysts.

HISTOPATHOLOGY: Cysts.

DISCUSSION: Masses such as this with no indistinctness of their borders can be confidently interpreted as representing cysts. They are prone to occur in the central portion of the breast in small-breasted women as in this case.

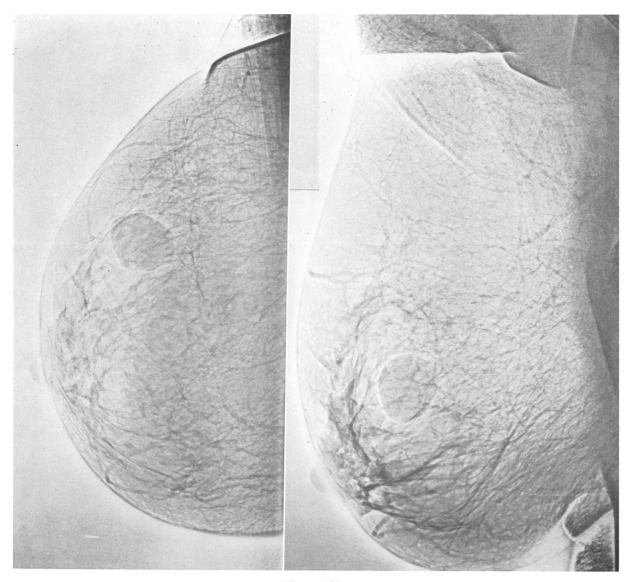

Figure 57.

HISTORY: A sixty-eight-year-old, nulliparous woman had thickening palpable in both breasts and a clinical impression of benign disease.

RADIOGRAPHIC OBSERVATIONS: The breasts were judged to be essentially normal in their appearance with the exception of a mass in the upper axillary quadrant of the breast. The margin of the mass was extremely sharp.

IMPRESSION: Cyst.

HISTOPATHOLOGY: Cyst.

DISCUSSION: A sharply limited mass with this configuration poses a problem in diagnosis. It is almost always a cyst. Occasionally a fibroadenoma will have a similar appearance.

A reexamination after three or four months should be done unless an aspiration or biopsy is carried out immediately.

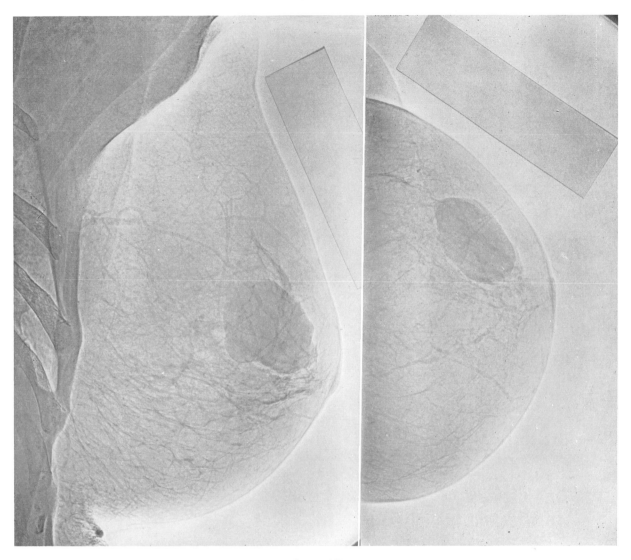

Figure 58.

HISTORY: A fifty-one-year-old, gravida 1 woman had a biopsy of the right breast four years before and now has slight thickening palpable in both breasts and a clinical impression of benign disease.

RADIOGRAPHIC OBSERVATIONS: The mass illustrated was in the right breast. It was somewhat lobulated with an extremely sharp margin. No evidence of invasion could be identified.

IMPRESSION: Cyst.

HISTOPATHOLOGY: Cyst.

DISCUSSION: There were bilateral masses—the one illustrated was in the right breast. There were three smaller, similar appearing masses on the left side. Although the illustrated mass is somewhat lobulated, the age of the patient and the influence of the observations on the left side led to a diagnosis of cystic disease rather than fibroadenoma and that reasoning proved to be correct.

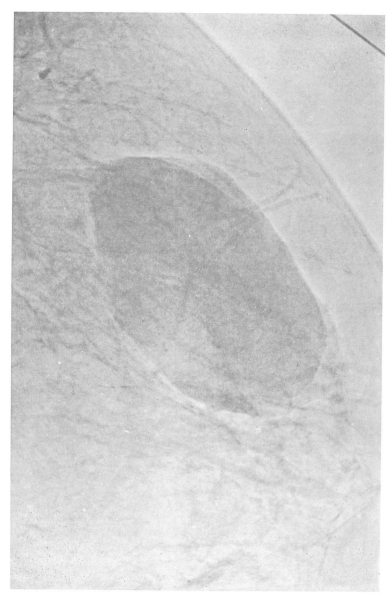

Figure 58 C *(Continued)*

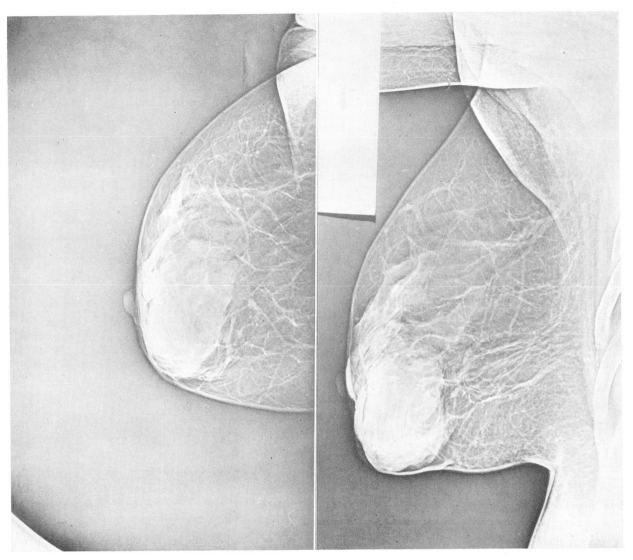

Figure 59.

HISTORY: A forty-five-year-old, gravida 4 woman discovered a mass behind the left nipple.

RADIOGRAPHIC OBSERVATIONS: The breast was noted to be composed mainly of fat. A superficially placed mass, that bulged but did not change the skin, was observed. Definite evidence of a carcinoma of the breast was not seen.

IMPRESSION: Cyst, left breast.

HISTOPATHOLOGY: Cyst.

DISCUSSION: The case can be interpreted rather confidently as a benign tumor because of its superficial location and its bulging. The skin remained unchanged. The margin of the mass, however, is not as sharp as one would like for a very firm impression of benign disease, so it was suggested in the X-ray report that the patient be followed if the tumor was not aspirated. The changes of the mass representing a carcinoma, however, were considered very slight.

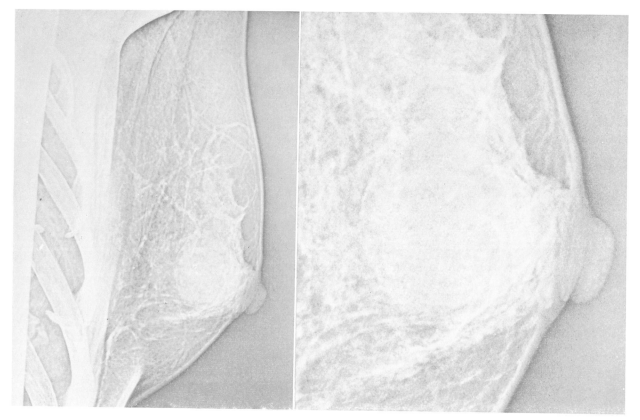

Figure 60.

HISTORY: A forty-nine-year-old, nulliparous woman had a history of multiple masses in both breasts and a number of previous biopsies. Three weeks before this examination she discovered a new mass which enlarged rapidly.

RADIOGRAPHIC OBSERVATIONS: The breasts were noted to be involved with some degree of mammary dysplasia. The mass was evident and located slightly to the axillary side of the nipple. On the lateral projection, part of the posterior wall was visible and some segments were rather sharp. Many segments of the wall seen on the caudal projection appeared very sharp.

IMPRESSION: Cyst.

HISTOPATHOLOGY: Cyst.

DISCUSSION: The case seems rather straightforward. The woman has had numerous biopsies for cysts in the past, she has the typical history of a rapidly enlarging mass, and the radiographic features are basically those of a benign tumor. The possibility that the mass represents a circumscribed carcinoma should be entertained, but the chances are very remote. Aspiration of the cyst could have been an ideal method of diagnosis and treatment.

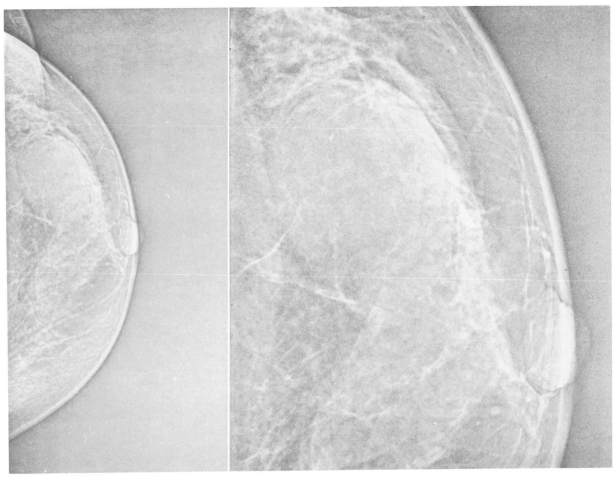

Figure 60 C-D *(Continued)*

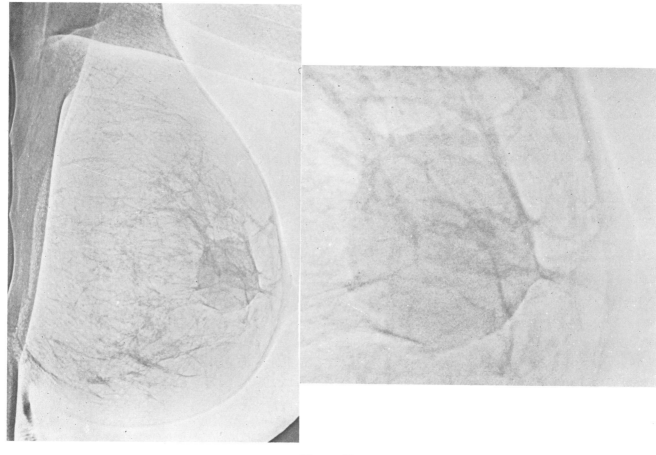

Figure 61.

HISTORY: A forty-one-year-old woman found a palpable mass in the right breast. The clinical impression was indeterminate.

RADIOGRAPHIC OBSERVATIONS: The breast was noted to be composed mainly of fat and, on this basis, was considered as a low-risk for breast cancer.

The rather superficial placement of the mass suggested benign disease. The margin, however, was not perfectly sharp and distinct, so the possibility of carcinoma had to be considered.

IMPRESSION: Suspicion of carcinoma.

HISTOPATHOLOGY: Cyst with hemorrhage.

DISCUSSION: In a case like this, aspiration greatly benefits diagnosis. The breast's parenchyma is of the type in which breast carcinoma does not often occur. The mass is superficially placed which is more in keeping with a benign tumor rather than a malignant one. There is no definite evidence of carcinoma, that is, the wall is not nodular and no spiculation nor calcifications are seen. Although the bulk of the evidence favors benign disease, one cannot simply rest on that diagnosis. The tumor should be aspirated or removed. To follow a tumor of this kind with repeat examinations is the *least* desirable form of treatment.

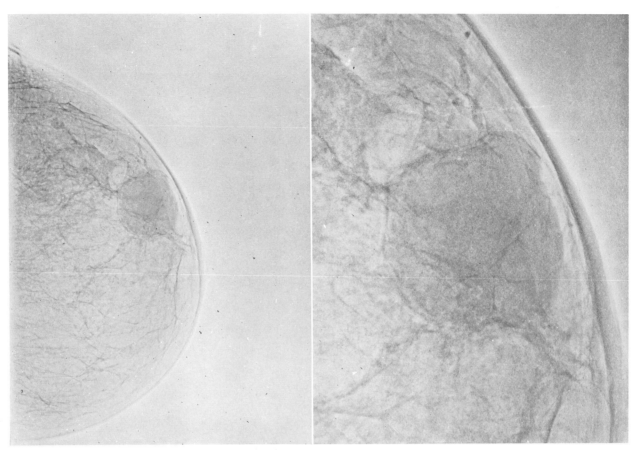

Figure 61 C-D *(Continued)*

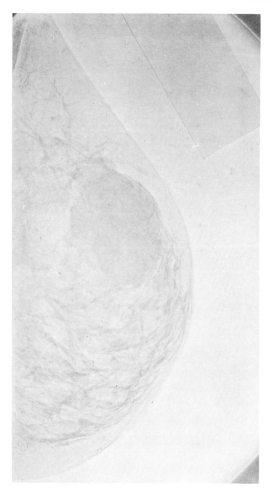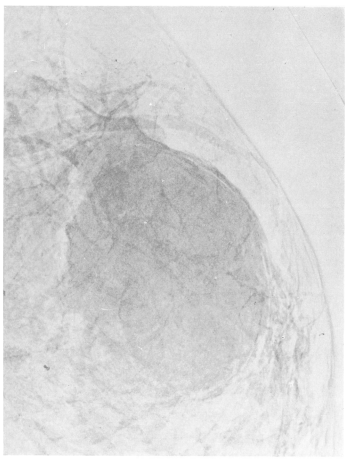

Figure 62.

HISTORY: A forty-three-year-old, gravida 5 woman who had had a biopsy of the left breast five years earlier, discovered a mass of several weeks duration in her breast.

RADIOGRAPHIC OBSERVATIONS: The breast was noted to be essentially normal in its overall appearance. Because of its rather sharp anterior border, the mass was thought most likely to represent a cyst, or as an outside possibility, a circumscribed form of carcinoma.

IMPRESSION: Large cyst.

HISTOPATHOLOGY: Cyst.

DISCUSSION: Tumors like this one, readily palpable and historically of short duration, are almost always cysts. Rarely do they represent circumscribed forms of carcinoma. It would seem that cyst aspiration would be an excellent method of diagnosis and treatment of this patient.

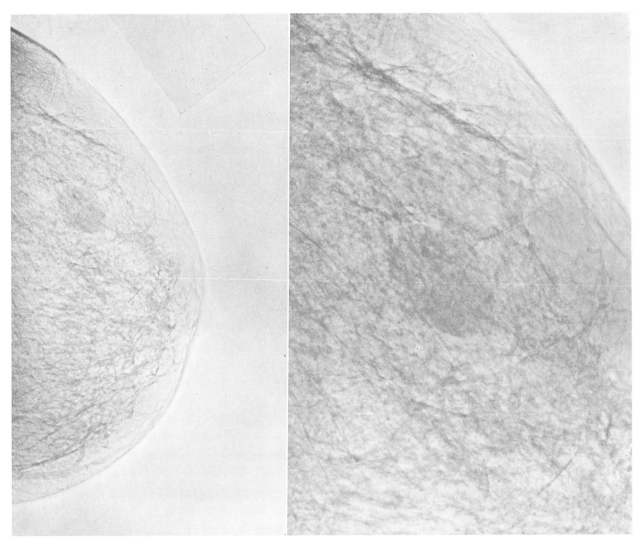

Figure 63.

HISTORY: A fifty-one-year-old, gravida 2 woman discovered a mass in the outer quadrant of her right breast. The clinical impression was indeterminate.

RADIOGRAPHIC OBSERVATIONS: Both breasts were symmetrically involved with a prominent duct pattern. A mass was observed in the outer quadrant of the right breast with an indistinct, irregular margin. At no point was its margin perfectly sharp. No nodularity could be identified.

IMPRESSION: Suspicion of medullary carcinoma with a differential diagnosis of cyst.

HISTOPATHOLOGY: Cyst.

DISCUSSION: It is very difficult to come to a correct diagnosis in a patient such as this. To begin with, the patient is fifty-one years of age and has a moderately severe prominent duct pattern. The mass is not perfectly outlined along any segment of its margin, although the breast is not so dense as to obscure it. Because of this apparent indistinctness of contour, the incorrect diagnosis of malignancy is unavoidable.

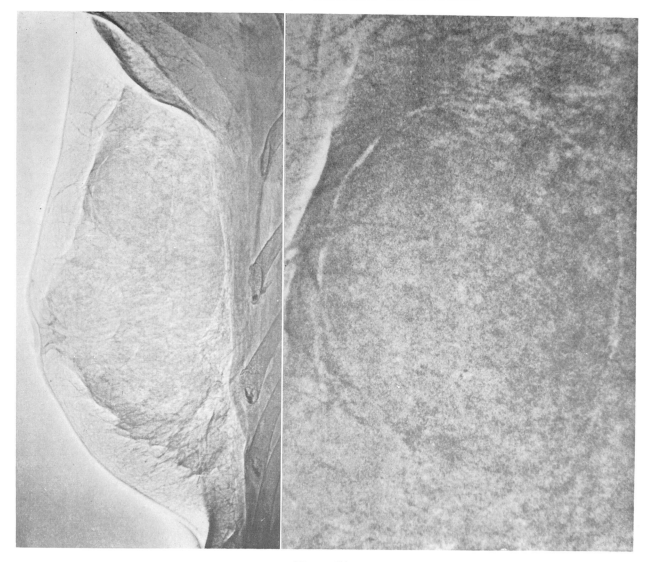

Figure 64.

HISTORY: A forty-four-year-old, nulliparous woman who has had three previous biopsies in each breast now complains of thickening in both breasts.

RADIOGRAPHIC OBSERVATIONS: The breasts were noted to be involved severely with a prominent duct pattern and what was interpreted as adenosis. The main observation concerned the mass in the upper portion of one breast. The margin of the mass, clearly visible around four fifths of its circumference, was sharply distinct.

IMPRESSION: Cyst.

HISTOPATHOLOGY: Cyst.

DISCUSSION: The radiographic report indicated that the most likely diagnosis in this patient was a cyst. It was recommended, however, that if aspiration or excision were not performed, the patient should be followed carefully by physical and radiographic examinations. The impression was influenced certainly by the ablty to see nearly all of the margin of the mass and also by the past history of this patient for cyst development.

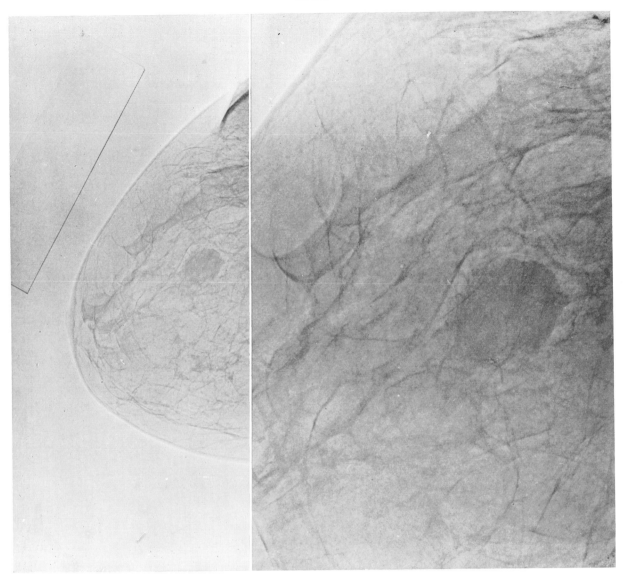

Figure 65.

HISTORY: A thirty-three-year-old, gravida 4 woman who had a biopsy of the left breast fourteen years before and now has a mass palpable in the upper portion on the left side.

RADIOGRAPHIC OBSERVATIONS: The general appearance of both breasts was not remarkable and they were thought to be essentially normal.

The chief observation concerned the mass. Note that its border appears slightly nodular in one projection and very indistinct in the other.

IMPRESSION: Possible medullary carcinoma.

HISTOPATHOLOGY: Cyst.

DISCUSSION: It is impossible to avoid an error such as this when the margin of the mass in two projections is demonstrated to be quite irregular and in some projections nodular.

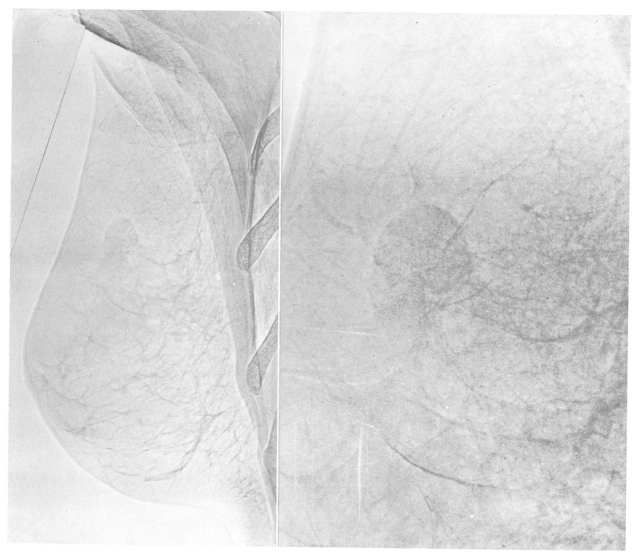

Figure 65 C-D *(Continued)*

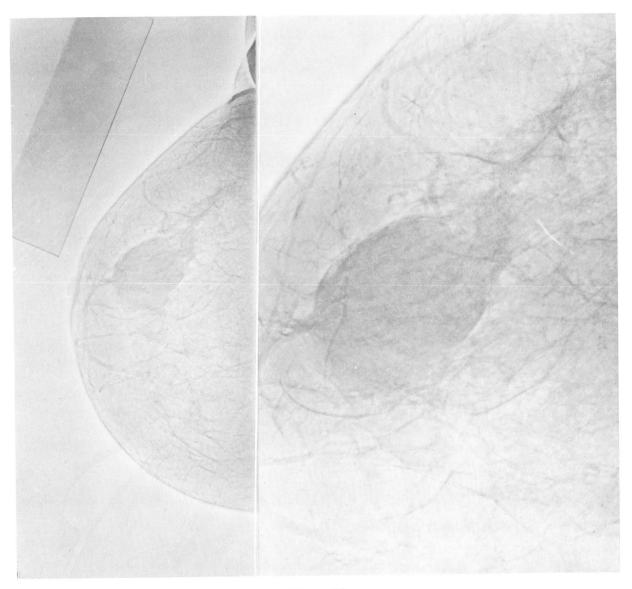

Figure 66.

HISTORY: A fifty-one-year-old, gravida 5 woman had a mass palpable in the left breast and a clinical impression of benign disease.

RADIOGRAPHIC OBSERVATIONS: The general appearance of both breasts was essentially normal.

The chief observation concerned the mass observed more or less in the central portion of the breast. Although some segments of its margin were very sharp on the caudal projection, others appeared rather indistinct especially on the lateral, posteriorly. Also, the anterior pole tended to be somewhat tapered.

IMPRESSION: Medullary carcinoma.

HISTOPATHOLOGY: Cyst.

DISCUSSION: Medullary carcinomas are very difficult to diagnose; only about 50 percent accuracy can be expected. They are most often confused with cysts as in this example.

It would probably be better to recommend aspiration of the tumor as the first method of treatment and if it could not be aspirated, then excision would be in order.

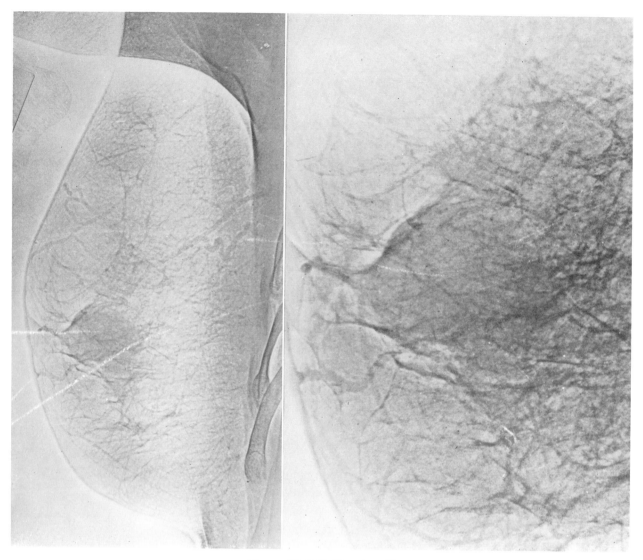

Figure 66 C-D *(Continued)*

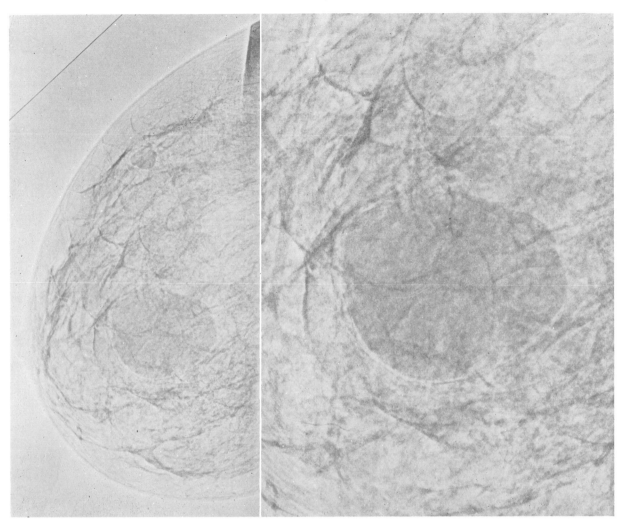

Figure 67.

HISTORY: A thirty-year-old, gravida 2 woman had a mass palpable in the left breast and a clinical impression of benign disease.

RADIOGRAPHIC OBSERVATIONS: The breast was considered essentially normal except for the masses. Note that there were two masses, one posterior to the nipple and a smaller one far to the axillary side. Their margins were very sharp, and in some areas there was a radiolucent halo. There were also two very small masses in the right breast.

IMPRESSION: Multiple cysts.

HISTOPATHOLOGY: Cysts.

DISCUSSION: Very frequently, multiple masses in both breasts represent either cysts or fibroadenomas. In this case, the age of the patient, the pattern of the breast tissue and the appearance of the contours of the masses strengthened the impression of benign disease. The larger mass was the key to diagnosis: It was judged benign because of its very sharp margin and radiolucent halo and determined to be a cyst because it lacks pronounced lobulation.

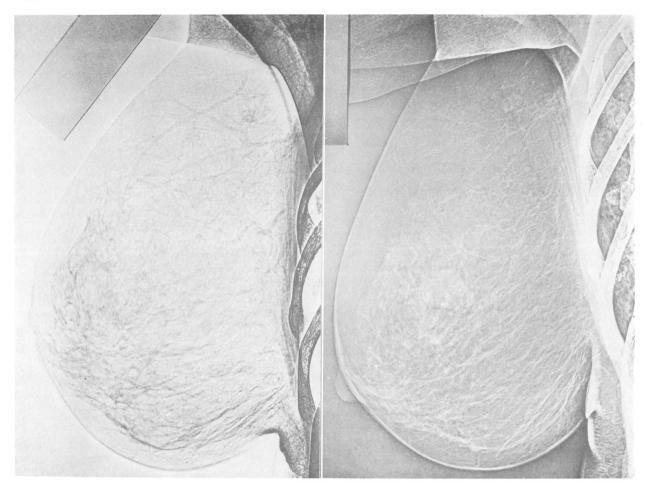

Figure 68.

HISTORY: A fifty-year-old, gravida 3 woman discovered a mass in her left breast.

RADIOGRAPHIC OBSERVATIONS: There were two examinations and they were separated by eighteen months. On the first study, the breast was noted to be involved with a prominent duct pattern of moderate severity.

On the second study, the well-circumscribed mass was identified. A radiolucent halo was seen around a portion of the periphery of the mass.

IMPRESSION: Cyst.

HISTOPATHOLOGY: Cyst.

DISCUSSION: Cysts characteristically can appear and disappear in very short intervals of time. The sharp margin of this tumor led one to believe that very likely it represented a benign tumor.

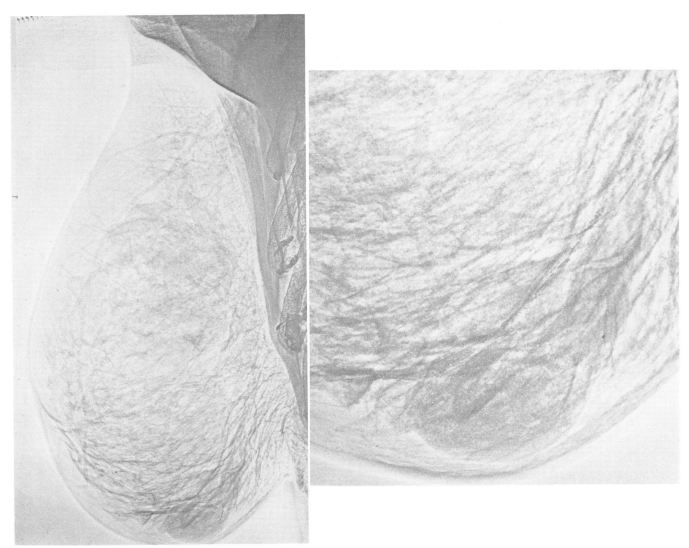

Figure 69.

HISTORY: A fifty-seven-year-old, gravida 1 woman had thickening palpable in both breasts and a mass on the left. The clinical impression was benign disease.

RADIOGRAPHIC OBSERVATIONS: A well-circumscribed, almost subcutaneous mass was observed. The failure to visualize the superior margin is attributed to overlying parenchymal densities rather than to any indistinctness to the margin of the mass.

IMPRESSION: Cyst.

HISTOPATHOLOGY: Cyst.

DISCUSSION: It is exceedingly unusual for a superficially placed mass such as this to represent a carcinoma. The location, in addition to the sharp margin of the mass, should lead one to a reasonable impression of a cyst.

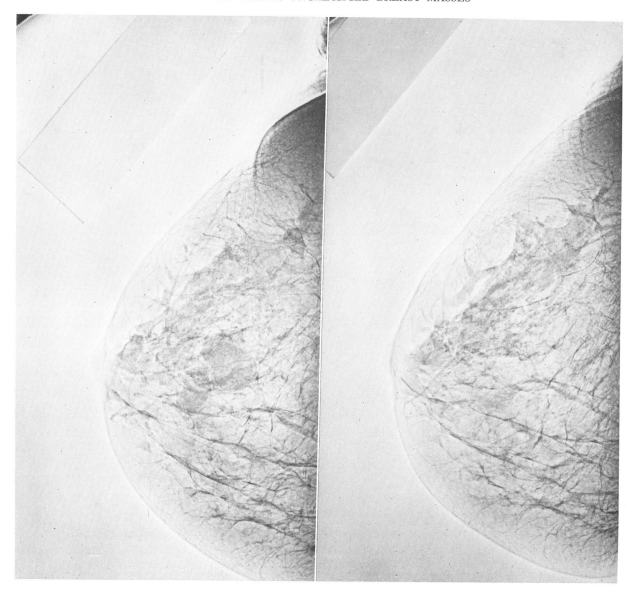

Figure 70.

HISTORY: A forty-eight-year-old, gravida 5 woman had masses palpable in both breasts (there were two examinations separated by ten weeks).

RADIOGRAPHIC OBSERVATIONS: The initial study, (A), revealed the breast to be involved with moderate amounts of mammary dysplasia. Two masses could be identified in the central portion. The margins of the masses were very sharp.

IMPRESSION: Cysts.

HISTOPATHOLOGY: None. Reexamination ten weeks later revealed complete disappearance of the masses.

DISCUSSION: Because it is not uncommon to see rapid fluctuation in the size and number of cysts, masses which are suspected of representing cysts should be reexamined after an interval of three months. In a large number of cases there will be an obvious change most frequently toward diminution in size or disappearance of the mass in question and appearance of others either in the opposite breast or in other areas of the same breast.

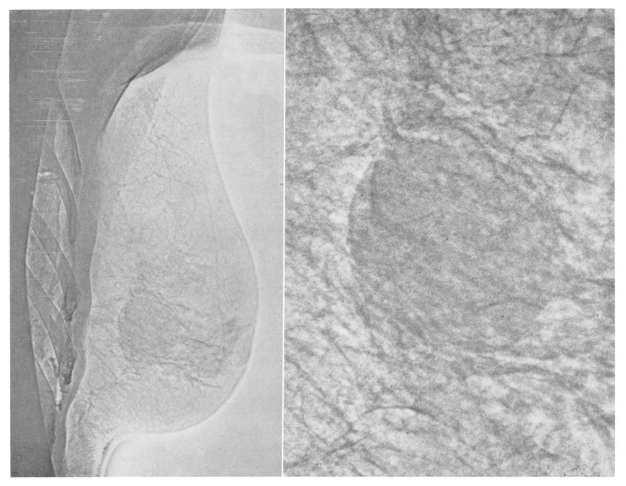

Figure 71.

HISTORY: A forty-three-year-old, gravida 1 woman had a biopsy of the right breast seven years before this examination. On physical examination she has masses in both breasts and a clinical impression of multiple cysts.

RADIOGRAPHIC OBSERVATIONS: Masses were observed in both breasts, the largest being on the right (A). The posterior margin of the mass was noted to be very sharp. The anterior margin was somewhat obscured by what is believed to be superimposition of other structures within the breast. The retracted nipple was seen but disregarded as it existed in both breasts.

IMPRESSION: Cyst.

HISTOPATHOLOGY: None.

DISCUSSION: It was recommended at the time of the original examination, (A), that if the mass was not aspirated or removed the patient be followed after a three-month interval. Follow-up examination, done four months later, (B), reveals marked spontaneous reduction in size of the cyst.

Of greater interest is the change in the appearance of the cyst when it became smaller. A diagnosis based on image (B) alone (of the second examination) would have been more toward malignancy. Note now that the margins at this time are much more irregular, especially posteriorly. The point, of course, is to demonstrate the value of serial examination of masses of which there is a strong opinion of cystic disease.

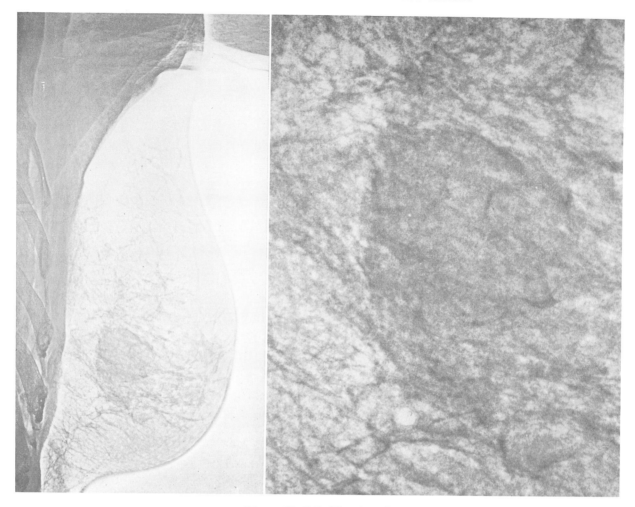

Figure 71 C-D *(Continued)*

ence of pregnancy and lactation, in which case they grow very rapidly only to regress after lactation has ceased.

Another consideration regarding cysts is the time at which the mammogram is done. If the cyst is distended with fluid, then we are likely to see a sharply contoured wall and arrive at a correct diagnosis of benign tumor. If, however, it is not distended (partially collapsed), the wall appears irregular and leads to a false diagnosis of carcinoma. This is why it is important to obtain mammography before aspiration. (Fig. 72)

Aspiration is a procedure to be recommended when the evidence for a cyst is predominant and a carcinoma entertained only as a very remote possibility. Some surgeons do not like to aspirate cysts for fear there may be a carcinoma arising in the wall of the cyst. This is a very rare form of carcinoma and, if it is present, the cyst's contents may provide a clue to the presence of the carcinoma by being sanguinous. There may also be abnormal cells that one can identify by Papanicolaou smear of the contents that are aspirated.

Finally, if there is a carcinoma within the cyst, the fluid typically will recur within a matter of a few weeks, whereas, if the mass represents a truly simple cyst, the fluid, if it recurs at all, does so over a much longer period of time. (Figs. 73, 74, 75, 76)

If the mass cannot be aspirated, then, of course, it must be excised, a needle biopsy performed, or the case must be followed very closely by repeat physical and radiographic examinations. This decision is dependent on many factors and must be individualized.

Follow-up radiographic examination immediately after removal of the cyst's contents probably is not necessary. If the preliminary radiographic impression was a benign tumor, likely a cyst, and if the physical findings were those of a cyst with the mass disappearing on aspiration, there is very little reason for immediate reexamination. If there is any doubt at all, then after removal of the cyst's contents, air can be injected and a double contrast image made which will show the wall of the cyst and any irregularity within it.

DIFFERENTIAL DIAGNOSIS OF CYST VERSUS FIBROADENOMA

It is of some interest to establish a differential diagnosis between a cyst and fibroadenoma. There are some features which permit a fairly accurate differential, and these can be seen in the following table. These are generalizations, but they can be useful guidelines.

Cyst versus Fibroadenoma

Cyst	*Fibroadenoma*
Middle age to elderly	Teenage to middle age
Round to oval	Lobulated
Associated dysplasia	Not as frequently associated with dysplasia
Not associated with pregnancy	Associated with pregnancy
Single or multiple	Single or multiple
Often bilateral	Not as frequently bilateral
Symmetrical involvement	Involvement not as asymmetrical

The age of the patient is of value in differential diagnosis, although there is considerable overlap. In general, fibroadenomas are much more common in teenagers and nulliparous twenty-year-olds. Cysts are more commonly found in slightly older women, whereas fibroadenomas in the older age groups tend to be calcified and are simple to diagnose.

The shape is important. A fibroadenoma, of course, has a tendency to be lobulated, while a cyst tends to be rather oval or round, although at times they can give somewhat of a lobulated appearance. In the author's experience, sharply contoured, lobulated tumors in the breast of pregnant or lactating women are always lactating adenomas.

The breasts generally are more severely dysplastic in women with cystic disease as opposed to the breasts of women with fibroadenomas. As mentioned, cysts are more commonly bilateral and symmetrical in their distribution than fibroadenomas which, if bilateral, tend to be asymmetrical.

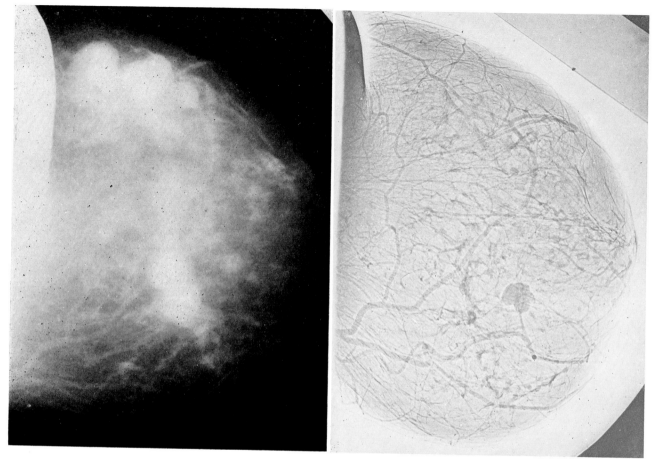

Figure 72.

HISTORY: A fifty-five-year-old, gravida 2 woman had on the initial study, (A), multiple masses palpable in her breasts and a clinical impression of benign disease. At the time of the follow-up study, (B), three years later, the clinical impression was the same.

RADIOGRAPHIC OBSERVATIONS: The multiple masses were seen within the breast, (A), and they were noted to have sharp margins. Radiographic evidence of a carcinoma could not be identified.

Follow-up examination revealed marked diminution in size of one of the masses and complete disappearance of the others.

IMPRESSION: Cystic disease.

HISTOPATHOLOGY: None.

DISCUSSION: The case illustrates the fluctuation that is quite characteristic of cystic disease. No biopsies or aspirations were performed. Often, as the patient grows older, the cystic disease tends to become less severe.

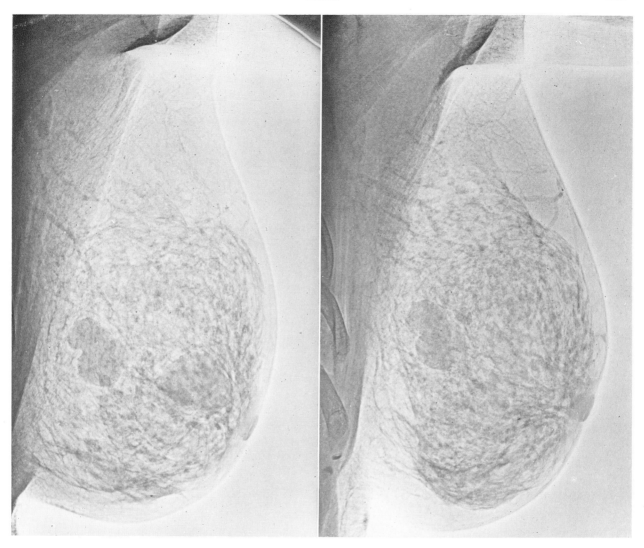

Figure 73.

HISTORY: A forty-eight-year-old, nulliparous woman had masses palpable in the left breast and a clinical impression of benign disease.

RADIOGRAPHIC OBSERVATIONS: Both breasts were severely involved with a prominent duct pattern. The first examination, (A), revealed two masses. The margins of the masses were somewhat sharp, without good evidence of a carcinoma.

IMPRESSION: Cyst.

HISTOPATHOLOGY: None.

DISCUSSION: Aspiration of the more anterior cyst yielded clear fluid. A repeat examination, after puncture, showed that the mass had disappeared. The case is considered incomplete in that the second mass was not treated. Because of its rather marked lobularity, certainly it should be aspirated, excised, or followed closely by repeat examinations.

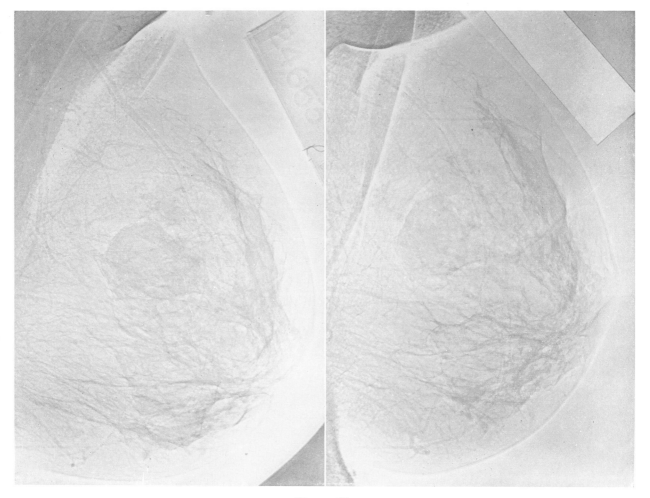

Figure 74.

HISTORY: A forty-seven-year-old, gravida 3 woman had masses palpable in both breasts. There were two examinations separated by six months. A cyst aspiration was performed in the interim.

RADIOGRAPHIC OBSERVATIONS: The breasts were noted to be involved with minor degrees of dysplasia. Note the mass in the axillary portion of the breast, (A). Its sharply contoured posterior and medial walls were seen and no evidence of malignancy could be identified. On the repeat examination after aspiration the mass was nearly completely gone, (B).

IMPRESSION: Cyst.

HISTOPATHOLOGY. None.

DISCUSSION: This is the type of mass that radiologists should encourage the referring physician to aspirate. All of the radiographic features of the mass are those of a cyst as well as the physical findings. Nothing is seen on the images to direct the diagnosis toward a carcinoma.

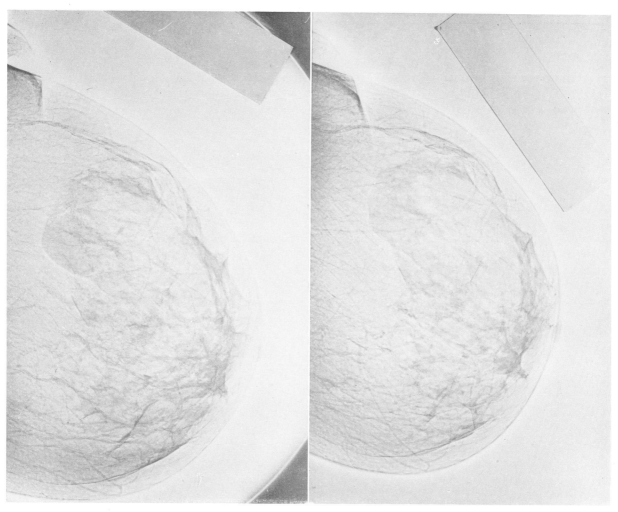

Figure 74 C-D *(Continued)*

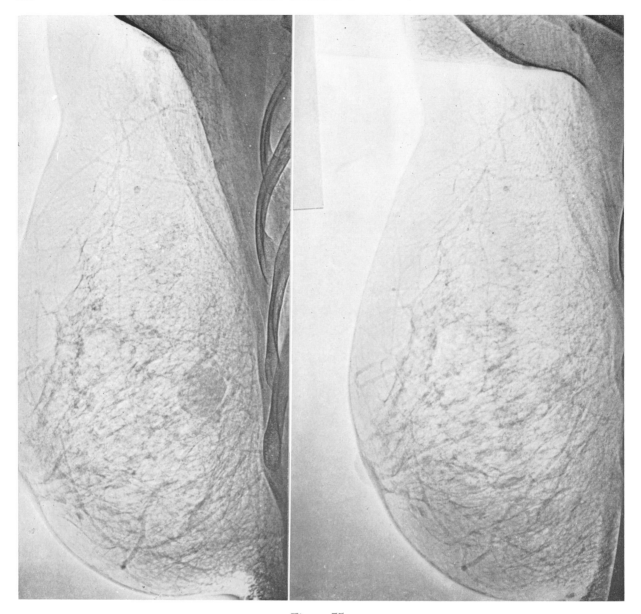

Figure 75.

HISTORY: A fifty-four-year-old, gravida 3 woman had a palpable mass in the axillary half of the left breast and a clinical impression of benign disease.

RADIOGRAPHIC OBSERVATIONS: Both breasts were noted to be involved with minor degrees of a prominent duct pattern. A 2 cm mass on the left was readily identified and its margin was extremely sharp in both projections. The general shape of the mass is oval to round, (A).

Follow-up examination, three months later, revealed complete disappearance without treatment, (B).

IMPRESSION: Cyst.

HISTOPATHOLOGY: Cyst.

DISCUSSION: The sharpness of the margin of the mass and the age of the patient permits a reasonable impression of a benign tumor, most likely a cyst. It would be unusual if it represented a fibroadenoma. Although the evidence for cyst is rather strong, it is considered essential to obtain a follow-up examination in three months unless the mass is aspirated or excised.

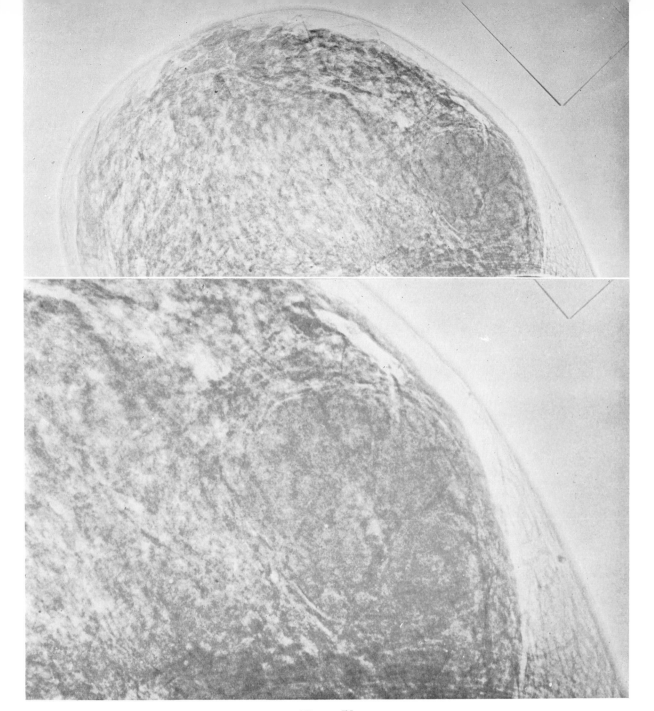

Figure 76.

HISTORY: A forty-four-year-old woman discovered a mass in the breast. The clinical impression was benign disease.

RADIOGRAPHIC OBSERVATIONS: Both breasts were involved severely with a prominent duct pattern.

A mass far to the axillary side was observed. Sharp segments of its margin could be identified, but the complete margin was not seen. The tumor was noted to be located very superfically.

IMPRESSION: Cyst with the recommendation that it be aspirated and, if not aspirated or excised, to be followed by repeat examination in three months.

HISTOPATHOLOGY: Cyst.

DISCUSSION: Not all of the margins of the mass can be identified. However, those segments which are seen are extremely sharp. That observation, together with the superficial location of the tumor and its general contour, led one to the impression of a simple cyst.

There should be some caution, however, as the breast is involved severely with a prominent duct pattern. Certainly, further diagnostic procedures must be done such as cyst aspiration or excision and, finally, as the last choice, a follow-up examination.

Chapter IX

Abscesses

ABSCESS ACCOUNTS for less than 1 percent of the uncalcified breast masses. Considering the great number of discrete masses within the breast, abscess is relatively important. There are two types: *acute* and *chronic*. Here we are more concerned with the acute variety, but the characteristics of the chronic will be mentioned in passing.

The historical features and physical findings are absolutely essential, since the radiographic features often simulate precisely those of a carcinoma. Even with all available information, it is sometimes impossible to make the correct diagnosis. Most abscesses occur in the lactating young woman. The patient is usually two to three days postpartum and will complain of a very tender, painful mass in the breast. Often there will be fever and chills. As will be seen in the examples, however, not all of the acute abscesses occur in the lactating breast. When one finds an example in the older woman, very frequently it is overdiagnosed as a carcinoma.

The radiographic findings are those of a fairly well-circumscribed mass. It can be located anywhere within the breast. In the lactating breast, more often than not, it is large, at times 6 centimeters in diameter. In the older age group they tend to be smaller, usually 1 to 2 centimeters in diameter. In the very acute forms, especially those that accompany lactation, edema of the areola and skin are prone to occur and should not mislead one into the diagnosis of carcinoma. These observations must be judged in the light of all of the findings, especially those of the history and physical examination. Axillary lymphadenopathy has been frequently observed.

The acute abscesses usually subside quickly with antibiotic therapy. Although it is not often necessary, a repeat mammographic examination of the area in question after an interval of two weeks following treatment usually demonstrates its complete disappearance. (Figs. 77, 78, 79, 80, 81, 82, 83, 84, 85)

CHRONIC ABSCESS

The historical features, physical findings and radiographic observations in chronic breast abscesses are quite different. They are seen in not only the young woman, but often in the middle-aged one. There is usually a long history of biopsies, excisions and drainages. The skin of the breast is usually markedly deformed by the scarring as a result of the abscess and the previous surgery. At times small draining sinuses may be seen. The location of the chronic abscess is often subareolar as opposed to that of the acute abscess which may be anywhere within the breast.

Physical findings are those of an irregular, masslike density which is quite similar to the physical findings of a carcinoma.

Radiographic observations of chronic abscess are typified by irregular distortion of the architectural pattern of the breast. This distortion differs some-

what from that produced by carcinoma which is usually fairly regular or symmetrical. The subareolar location accompanied frequently by nipple retraction is also characteristic of chronic abscess. (Fig. 86)

Some notable exceptions to the usual chronic breast abscess include tuberculosis and some parasitic diseases. Tuberculosis, of course, is not a common disease in the United States now and, therefore, that type of abnormality of the breast is only infrequently observed. Where there is a high incidence of tuberculosis, however, involvement of the breast is quite common. Several cases of tuberculosis have been observed, and in only one of them was there a definite mass within the breast which was not calcified. It had an irregular margin and was diagnosed as very likely representing a carcinoma, perhaps of a medullary variety. It was

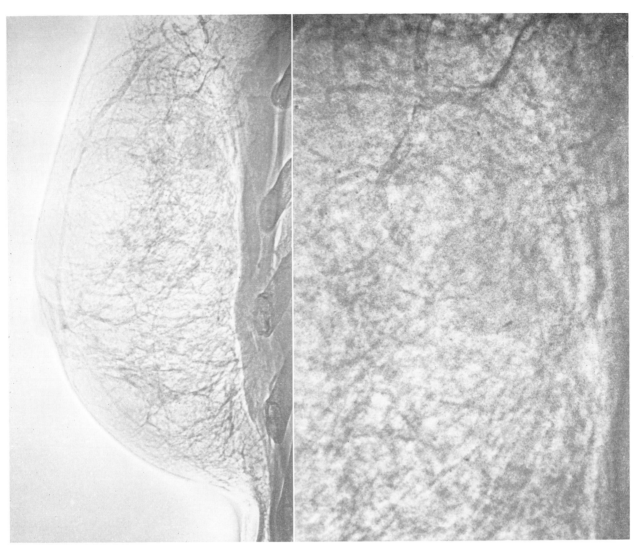

Figure 77.

HISTORY: A forty-nine-year-old, gravida 12 woman had a painful mass in the left breast and a past history of breast abscess.

RADIOGRAPHIC OBSERVATIONS: There is some slight degree of prominent duct pattern in both breasts but it was very minimal. The chief observation concerned the mass identified near the chest wall rather high in the left breast. The margins of the mass were noted to be indistinct and in some areas slightly nodular.

IMPRESSION: Carcinoma of the breast or breast abscess. It was recommended that the patient be reexamined after a short interval of antibiotic therapy.

HISTOPATHOLOGY: None.

DISCUSSION: Reexamination three weeks later revealed complete disappearance of the mass. If one considers the case only on the basis of the radiographic observations, a carcinoma of the breast would be the dominant opinion. The chances of being correct would be in the realm of 50 percent, with the balance of the cases being primarily cysts and, secondly, fibroadenomas.

With the consideration of the history of the patient, one can reasonably have a second impression of breast abscess and make a recommendation for treatment and a follow-up examination.

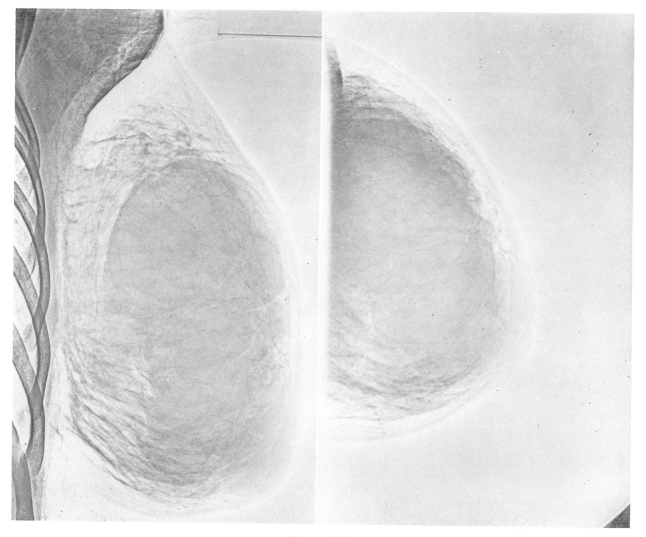

Figure 78.

HISTORY: A sixteen-year-old, gravida 2, three weeks postpartum had an extremely tender and painful mass palpable in the right breast.

RADIOGRAPHIC OBSERVATIONS: A large mass in the upper portion of the right breast was observed, with edema of the areola and skin. It had a rather sharp superior and posterior delineation.

IMPRESSION: Breast abscess.

HISTOPATHOLOGY: Breast abscess.

DISCUSSION: Recent pregnancy and complaints of severe pain and tenderness in the area of abnormality are important factors in this diagnosis. Also, there is no clear evidence of carcinoma, that is, there are no calcifications nor areas of spiculation. A diffuse carcinoma of the breast producing edema of the skin and areola usually does not form such a well-demarcated mass.

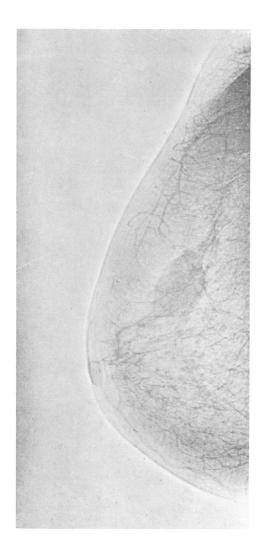
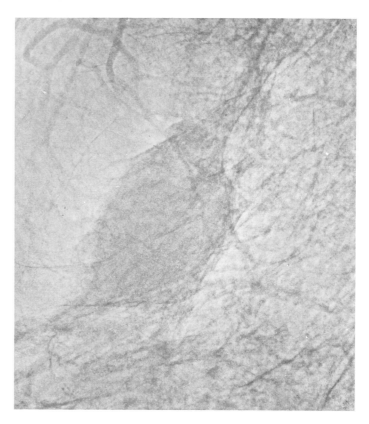

Figure 79.

HISTORY: A fifty-one-year-old, gravida 6 woman complained of a painful swelling in the left breast.

RADIOGRAPHIC OBSERVATIONS: Both breasts were noted to be composed mainly of fat and considered essentially normal.

The chief observation concerned the mass which was noted to have a very irregular border with some tapering of the anterior and posterior pole.

IMPRESSION: Possible carcinoma but in view of the history, a breast abscess was considered.

HISTOPATHOLOGY: Chronic breast abscess.

DISCUSSION: A consideration of the mass alone would lead one to a rather strong impression of a carcinoma with the expectation of being correct in that diagnosis about 50 percent of the time. When the physical findings and the history were considered, then a breast abscess became a dominant impression with the recommendation that the patient be placed on antibiotic therapy and reexamined after a short interval.

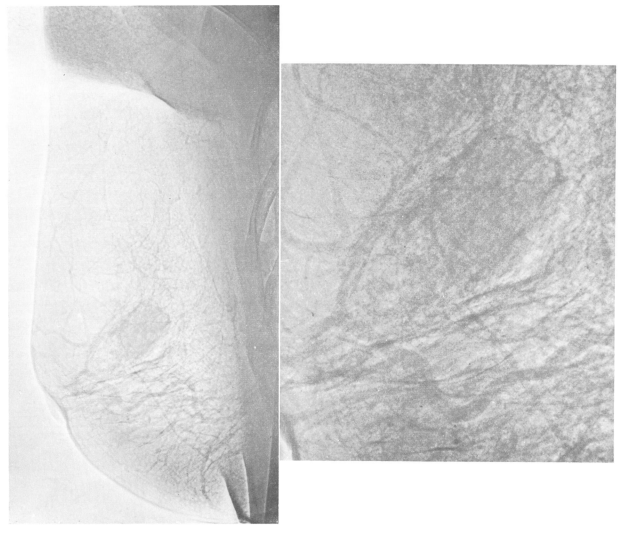

Figure 79 C-D *(Continued)*

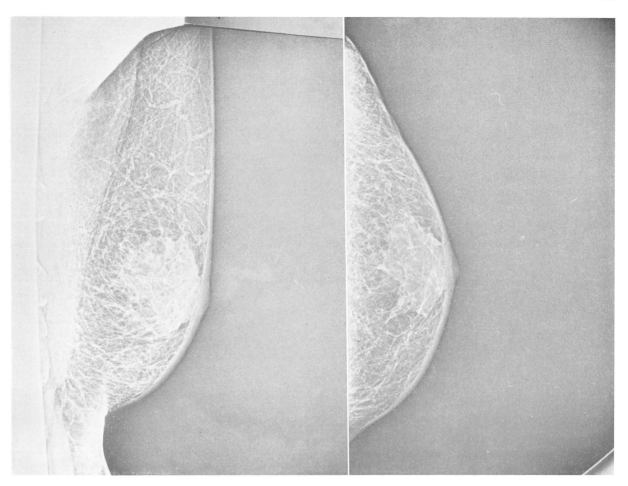

Figure 80.

HISTORY: A sixty-one-year-old man had a painful, tender breast with recent enlarge-ment and a palpable mass in the central portion. The clinical impression was of inflam-matory disease.

RADIOGRAPHIC OBSERVATIONS: The mass observed beneath the breast was noted to be very irregular. The opposite breast in this patient was involved with very minor degrees of gynecomastia with significant edema of the areola and the skin of the breast.

IMPRESSION: Carcinoma of the male breast with an outside possibility of breast abscess because of the physical findings and the history.

HISTOPATHOLOGY: Breast abscess.

DISCUSSION: This case is considered extremely unusual and it demonstrates the in-ability of the radiologist to come to a reasonable impression without consideration of the clinical symptoms and the physical findings.

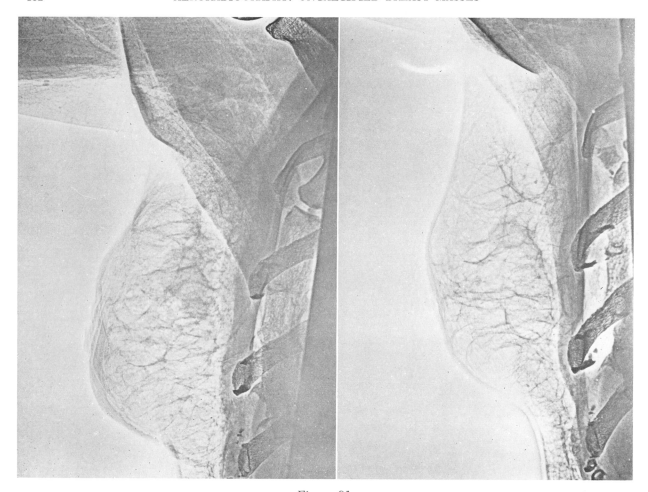

Figure 81.

HISTORY: A thirty-nine-year-old, gravida 5 woman discovered a mass in her left breast that was slightly tender to palpation. It did not have characteristics of a carcinoma on physical examination. The clinical impression was breast abscess. The patient returned for a follow-up examination two months later after antibiotic therapy.

RADIOGRAPHIC OBSERVATIONS: On the initial study it was felt rather strongly that the patient had a carcinoma. One can identify readily an indistinct mass in the upper portion of the left breast with thickening of the areolar shadow and of the skin over the lower portion of the breast. In addition, multiple lymph nodes are seen in the axilla, (A).

On the repeat study after antibiotic therapy, all of these changes disappeared, (B).

IMPRESSION: Initially the mass was thought strongly to represent a carcinoma, an impression that was disproved by the repeat examination.

HISTOPATHOLOGY: None.

DISCUSSION: A mass of this type cannot be correctly identified on the basis of radiographic evidence alone. Often an abscess is accompanied by regional lymphadenopathy and thickening of the skin, both good indicators of carcinoma. Fortunately, in this case, the characteristic physical findings determined the diagnosis, and after treatment, all signs and symptoms disappeared.

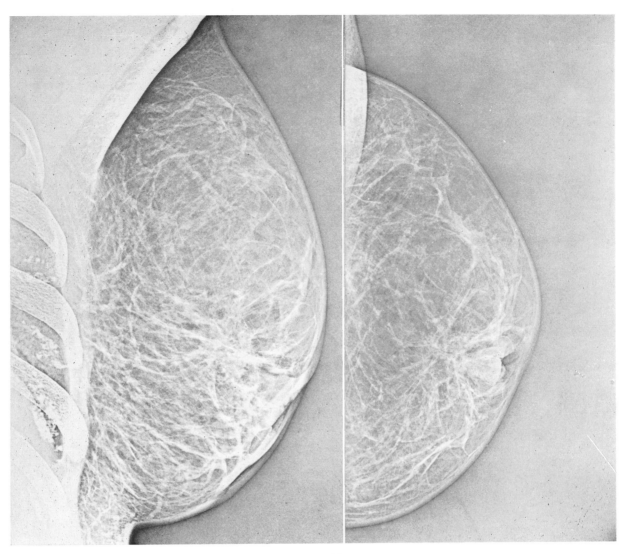

Figure 82.

HISTORY: A twenty-five-year-old, gravida 3 woman has had a history of breast abscess on the right side for two years and now complains of pain in the right breast.

RADIOGRAPHIC OBSERVATIONS: The marked distortion of the architecture of the breast in the subareolar area was considered somewhat characteristic for chronic breast abscess with scarring.

IMPRESSION: Scarring from chronic breast abscess.

HISTOPATHOLOGY: None.

DISCUSSION: The case has been followed for a long period of time and there has not been a change. The importance of the case is to caution the observer not to quickly make a diagnosis of carcinoma in the face of distortions such as these. The distortion is somewhat irregular, whereas the distortion produced by a carcinoma is usually somewhat "regular." Of equal importance is the history, and that must always be considered heavily.

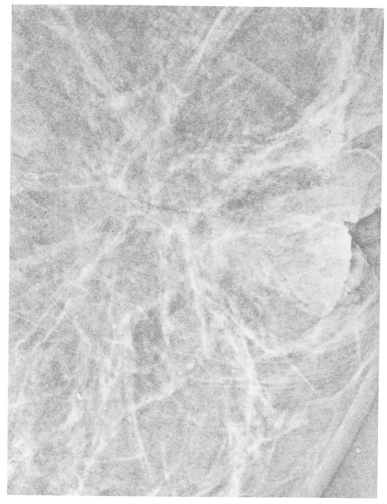

Figure 82 C *(Continued)*

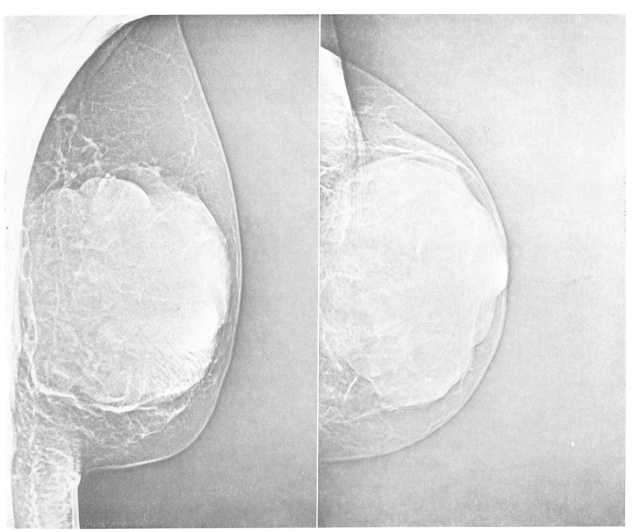

Figure 83.

HISTORY: A thirty-year-old, gravida 1 woman discovered a mass in her right breast which enlarged rapidly over a two-week period. She is a patient with chronic renal disease who has had a renal transplant and was receiving immunosuppressive drugs.

RADIOGRAPHIC OBSERVATIONS: A large mass in the right breast was readily observed. It appeared to be somewhat multilobulated. Its margins were rather sharp, there were no distinct areas of invasion nor were there calcifications. Apart from the mass, both breasts were considered normal. The radiographic impression was not confident.

IMPRESSION: Cystosarcoma phylloides, or some other form of sarcoma, with the added consideration of a multiloculated cyst.

HISTOPATHOLOGY: Breast abscess.

DISCUSSION: The patient had no fever or chills. The breast was only slightly tender and the mass felt somewhat cystic. Because of the historical features and the physical findings, the first impression was for cystosarcoma although the chances of being correct were rather minimal. The diagnosis of breast abscess was surprising in a patient with no systemic symptoms and perhaps is related to the fact that the patient was on immunosuppressive drugs.

characterized as a mass which did not have the usual features of either a benign tumor or carcinoma. (Fig. 87)

A separate issue is a very frequent, low-grade chronic inflammatory condition of the areola. It does not always present as a mass within the breast but often is associated with a mass-like density in the subareolar area. One should be very careful not to overdiagnose this condition as representing a carcinoma, perhaps of the Paget's variety. Typically, there is a history and physical finding of inflammatory disease, and these facts should influence the interpretation strongly. Also, the absence of other evidence of carcinoma, such as calcifications in the subareolar area to indicate the intraductal carcinoma accompanying a Paget's carcinoma, should dissuade one from diagnosing the abnormal inflammatory change of the areola, which is quite common, as the relatively rare form of carcinoma of Paget. (Fig. 88)

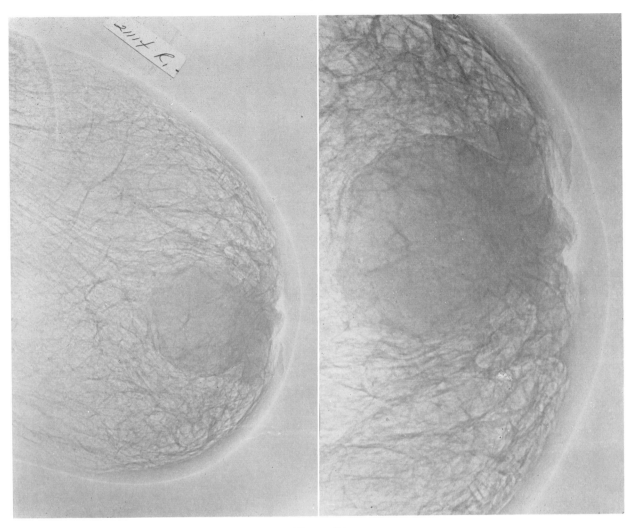

Figure 84.

HISTORY: A seventy-one-year-old, gravida 3 woman had a large palpable mass beneath the nipple of the right breast with reddening and edema of the skin. The clinical impression was inflammatory carcinoma.

RADIOGRAPHIC OBSERVATIONS: Both breasts were noted to be composed mainly of fat and essentially normal in their general appearance.

The chief observations concerned the mass beneath the nipple. In some areas the mass appeared rather irregular. Note that there is nipple retraction and marked edema of the skin.

IMPRESSION: Advanced carcinoma.

HISTOPATHOLOGY: Breast abscess.

DISCUSSION: An error such as this is impossible to avoid. The patient's age influences the radiographic impression. The likelihood of a breast abscess presented as a sharply circumscribed tumor such as this is so remote that one must always consider it as a carcinoma.

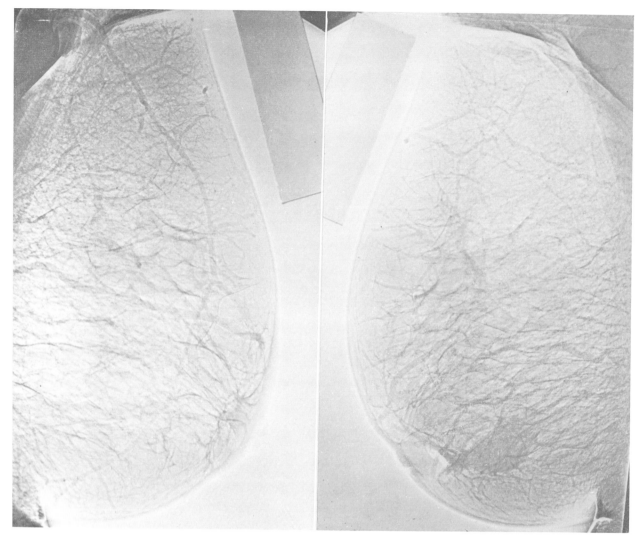

Figure 85.

HISTORY: A thirty-seven-year-old, nulliparous woman complained of redness of the skin of the breast and a mass in the subareolar area on the left side of one year's duration.

RADIOGRAPHIC OBSERVATIONS: A mass-like density with reaction of a portion of the skin was noted in the left breast. The margins of the mass were somewhat irregular. No clear evidence of a carcinoma could be identified.

IMPRESSION: Suspicion of carcinoma, left breast, but in view of the history and physical findings an abscess was also considered.

HISTOPATHOLOGY: Breast abscess.

DISCUSSION: The case is considered very difficult because of the poor delineation of the mass. Many of the margins are somewhat irregular and there is skin retraction.

The history and physical findings are valid to warrant a differential diagnosis between a carcinoma and an abscess.

The opposite breast exhibited typical areolar edema of low-grade inflammatory disease which is relatively common.

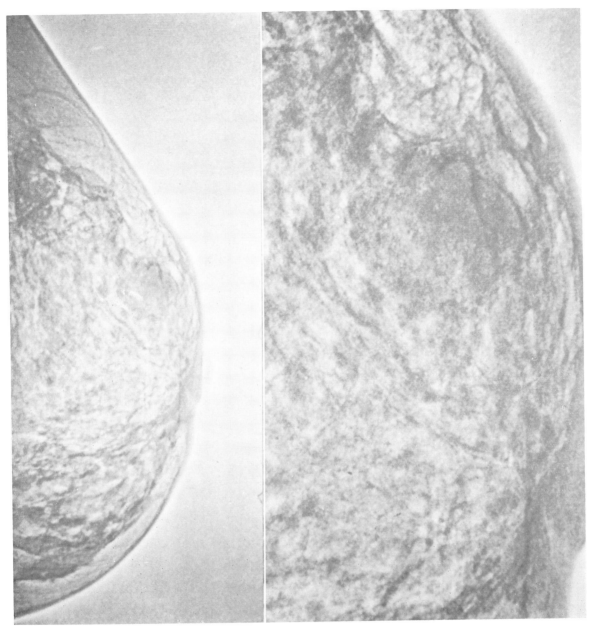

Figure 86.

HISTORY: A forty-five-year-old, gravida 1 woman complained of an infection in the left breast of two week's duration. The clinical impression was breast abscess.

RADIOGRAPHIC OBSERVATIONS: A mass located rather superficially in the sub-areolar area was identified. All of its margins could not be seen clearly and there was bulging and edema of the skin and subcutaneous areas.

IMPRESSION: Suspicion for carcinoma with an outside possibility of breast abscess.

HISTOPATHOLOGY: Breast abscess.

DISCUSSION: The case could be interpreted correctly by virtue of the history alone. However, it appeared at the time of the examination that the poorly limited mass producing bulging and an abnormality of the skin could also be due to a carcinoma. Such masses cannot be confidently interpreted as benign or malignant.

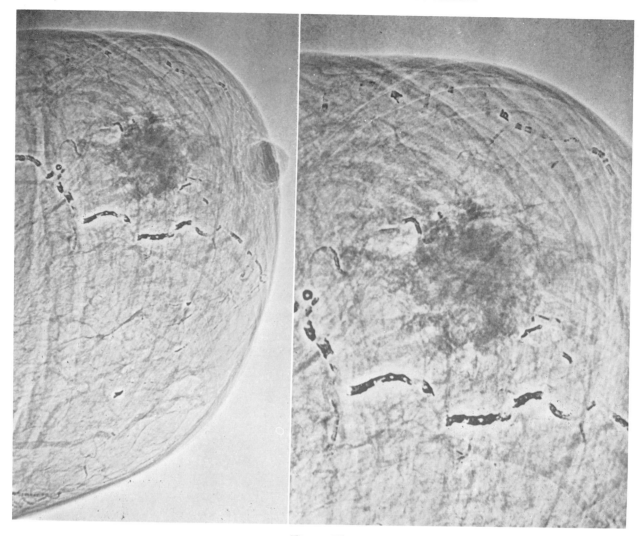

Figure 87.

HISTORY: An eighty-one-year-old, gravida 15 woman had had a mass in the left breast for one year and an orange-colored discharge from the left nipple.

RADIOGRAPHIC OBSERVATIONS: Both breasts were composed mainly of fat. The major observations concerned the mass. It was noted to be uncalcified and to have a rather irregular margin, somewhat nodular in areas.

IMPRESSION: Carcinoma of the breast.

HISTOPATHOLOGY: Tuberculosis.

DISCUSSION: The case is exceedingly unusual; it is one of an eighty-one-year-old woman with a palpable mass and radiographic observations consistent with carcinoma. One cannot escape the false positive diagnosis of carcinoma.

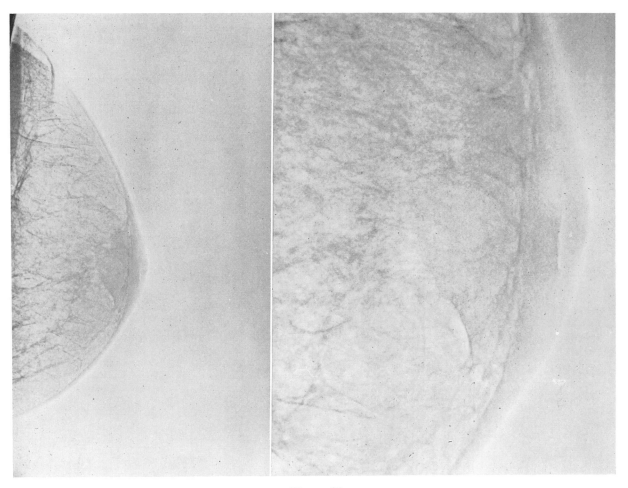

Figure 88.

HISTORY: A forty-one-year-old, gravida 2 woman had a clinical impression of inflammatory disease involving the right areola.

RADIOGRAPHIC OBSERVATIONS: (A) The thickening of the areolar shadow on one side was very apparent as the two breasts were compared. Note that the areola was discoid and presented as a mass in the subareolar area.

(B) Normal side for comparison. No evidence of a carcinoma could be identified. There were no calcifications.

IMPRESSION: Inflammatory disease of the areola.

HISTOPATHOLOGY: None.

DISCUSSION: The patient was treated with antibiotics and the inflammation subsided. The differential diagnosis concerns whether the areola thickening is due to carcinoma or inflammatory disease. To begin with, inflammatory disease is much more common than Paget's carcinoma. In addition, there is no other evidence of carcinoma. That is, there is no spiculated mass or tumor calcifications seen within the breasts to support the diagnosis of carcinoma. In addition, of course, is the very important physical finding of painful, red, swollen areola very consistent with infection.

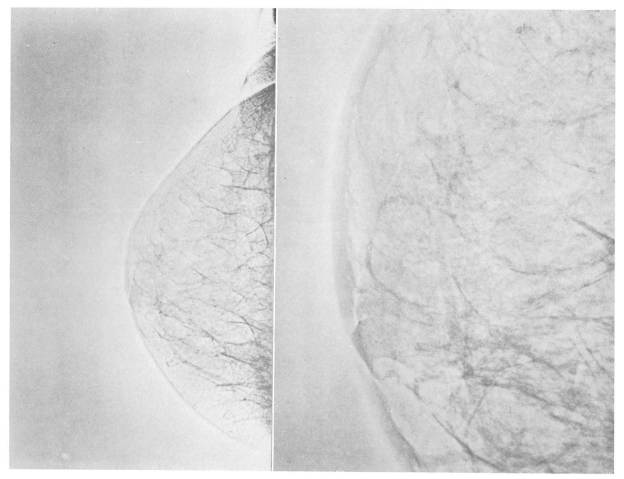

Figure 88 C-D *(Continued)*

Chapter X

Hematomas

THE SUBJECT OF HEMATOMA is an important consideration in the differential diagnosis of uncalcified breast masses. There is usually sufficient evidence to permit an accurate distinction between hematoma and carcinoma.

Here, again, the history is important. However, one must be very careful when presented with a patient who has had the following series of events: trauma to the breast, often an auto accident or a blow from a child, and then several days later, while palpating the tender area, discovery of a mass. Occasionally this is the first self-examination performed by the patient, and the palpated mass is a carcinoma which probably had been present for a considerable period of time prior to the trauma.

The radiographic features early in the course of the hematoma appear to be characteristic. There is usually a mass or group of masses at the site of the trauma and they are not sharply contoured. An important feature is that they do not have the usual features of malignancy. There is no spiculation or nodularity to their margins, and at the same time they do not have the features of the typical benign tumor: They are not lobulated, nor do they have a sharp contour. There may be edema of the skin and the subcutaneous area if the X-ray beam is tangential to the area of involvement. (Figs. 89, 90, 91, 92)

Another common hematoma is the one that occurs postoperatively. In one case, a woman underwent a biopsy for a mass within the breast, and some weeks after the biopsy discovered the mass to be even larger than before the operation. Her concern was that the surgeon might not have removed the area in question, and that it represented a carcinoma that had grown in the interim.

The radiographic features are characteristic. There will be a mass, typically in the subcutaneous area, often with a convex posterior border. One should diagnose confidently that it represents a hematoma. If there is any question at all, a follow-up examination after a few weeks usually reveals the disappearance of the mass and the appearance of typical scarring from previous biopsy. (Fig. 93)

If there is any question as to whether a particular mass represents a hematoma, a repeat examination after a few weeks will reveal its diminution in size at least and, at times, its complete disappearance.

The late features of hematoma are mainly calcifications and are not of concern in this presentation. Very briefly, in early stages they are eggshell calcifications, later on giving way to more densely calcified, but still somewhat spherical, masses.

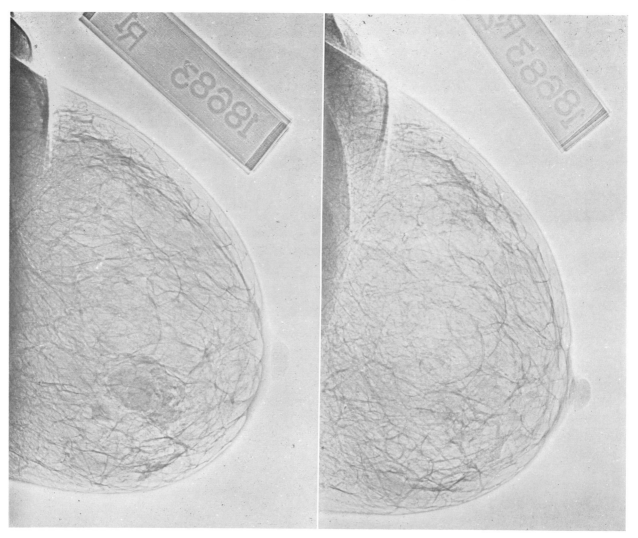

Figure 89.

HISTORY: A forty-two-year-old, gravida 5 woman injured her right breast in an automobile accident several days before the radiographic examination.

RADIOGRAPHIC OBSERVATIONS: Multiple, mass-like densities in the medial half of the right breast were observed. It was noted there was no clear evidence of carcinoma, that is, there was no spiculation and no tumor calcifications. At the same time the masses were not characterized as having the usual appearance of benign tumors.

IMPRESSION: Hematoma.

HISTOPATHOLOGY: None.

DISCUSSION: Follow-up examination made four weeks after the original study provides the evidence to substantiate the impression of hematoma. On the follow-up examination, one can observe very small, faint areas of lucency representing fat necrosis which eventually will calcify.

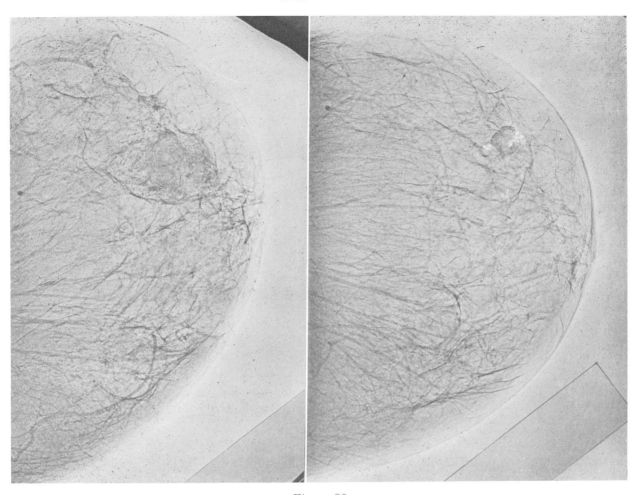

Figure 90.

HISTORY: A sixty-one-year-old, gravida 2 woman injured her breast one week before mammographic examination. Shortly after the injury, on palpating a tender area, she discovered a mass.

RADIOGRAPHIC OBSERVATIONS: There are two images of the left breast made at intervals of eight weeks. On the first were noted mass-like densities which did not have the usual features of either a benign or a malignant lesion and were somewhat characteristic of hematoma.

The second examination revealed marked reduction in the size of the mass which is now nonhomogeneous, perhaps representing a manifestation of fat necrosis which one would expect to eventually calcify.

IMPRESSION: Hematoma.

HISTOPATHOLOGY: None.

DISCUSSION: The case is considered quite characteristic for hematoma. Typically, the mass does not have the usual features of a benign or malignant lesion. Masses often present in a group. Follow-up examination after a short interval, of course, is invaluable.

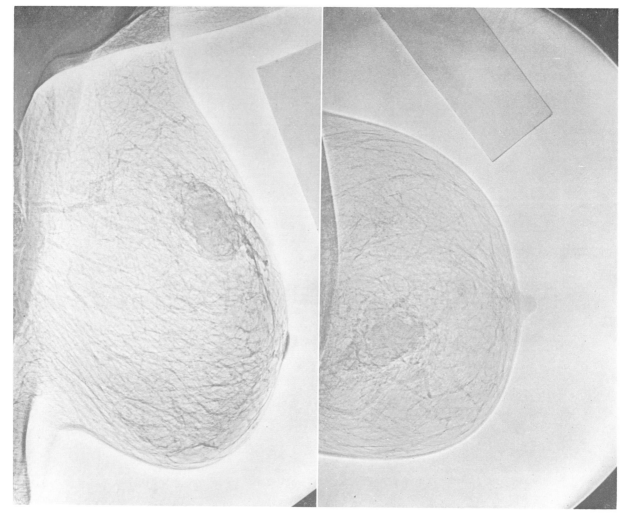

Figure 91.

HISTORY: A seventy-one-year-old, gravida 3 woman injured her right breast and several days later palpated a mass in that breast.

RADIOGRAPHIC OBSERVATIONS: The mass-like density was obvious. It was noted to be fairly limited and without good evidence of the usual carcinoma or benign tumor.

IMPRESSION: Hematoma.

HISTOPATHOLOGY: None.

DISCUSSION: A follow-up examination made several weeks later revealed almost complete disappearance of the mass. The case represents another instance of hematoma, characterized by history of trauma and a mass-like density that does not have the usual appearance of any commonly-encountered benign or malignant process.

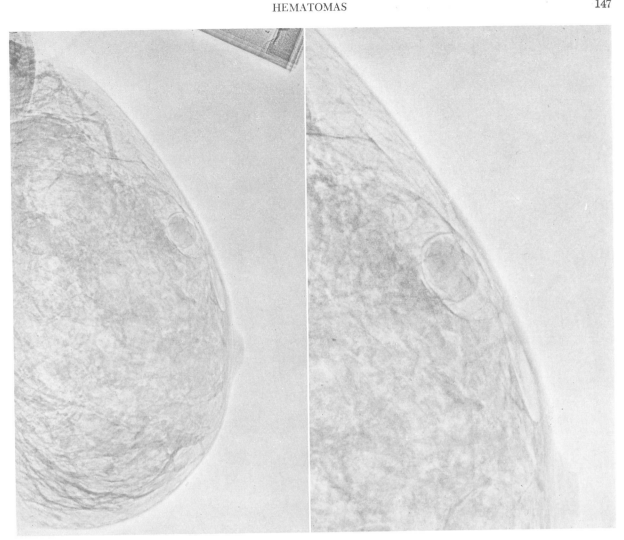

Figure 92.

HISTORY: A fifty-two-year-old, gravida 1 woman discovered a lump in her right breast in the upper axillary quadrant, the site of trauma two months before.

RADIOGRAPHIC OBSERVATIONS: A small subcutaneous mass in the right breast was observed. It was seen to have a very thin capsule with relative radiolucency, indicating some of the contents was fat and it had additional density of epithelial or connective tissue within the encapsulated area.

IMPRESSION: Benign tumor of the right breast, perhaps a lipoma.

HISTOPATHOLOGY: None.

DISCUSSION: The mass was not visible on the follow-up examination made four months after the original study. Its disappearance may indicate that it was related to trauma, possibly representing a hematoma that was later resorbed.

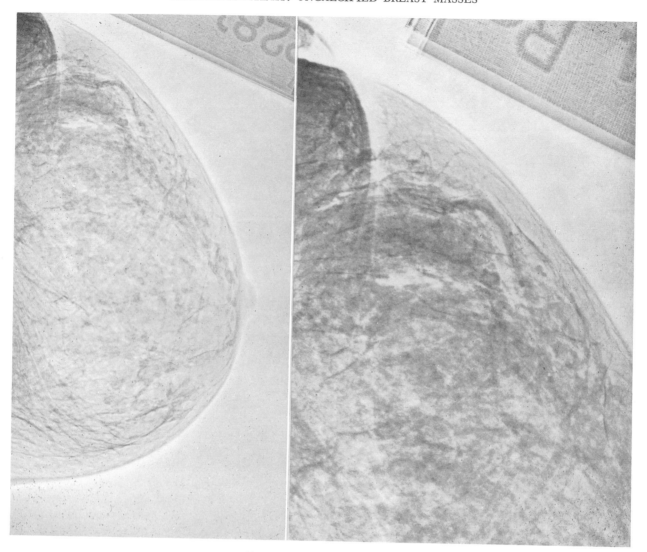

Figure 92 C-D *(Continued)*

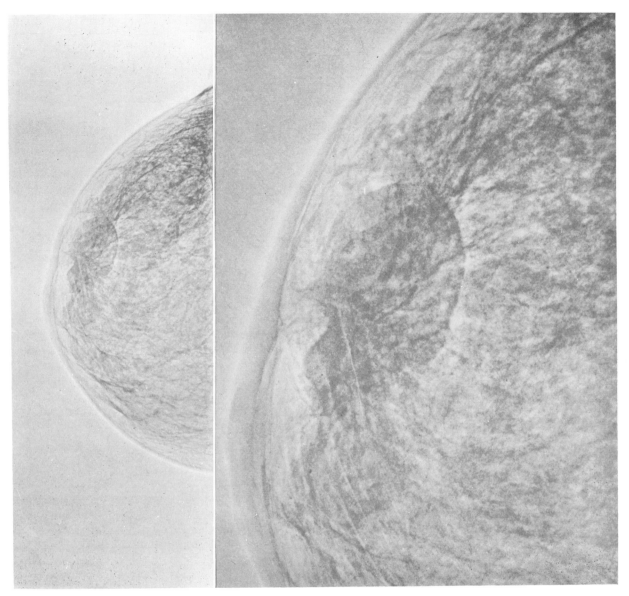

Figure 93.

HISTORY: A forty-five-year-old, gravida 2 woman had a biopsy of the left breast four weeks before the XR study. Three weeks later she discovered a mass at the site of the biopsy. The clinical impression was hematoma.

RADIOGRAPHIC OBSERVATIONS: A slight thickening of the skin and a subcutaneous mass with a very sharp posterior margin were observed. The breast was judged to be involved with mammary dyplasia.

IMPRESSION: Hematoma.

HISTOPATHOLOGY: None.

DISCUSSION: The follow-up examination, (B), made six months after the original study, confirmed the impression. Note the mass had disappeared nearly completely, and there is beginning retraction from scar formation.

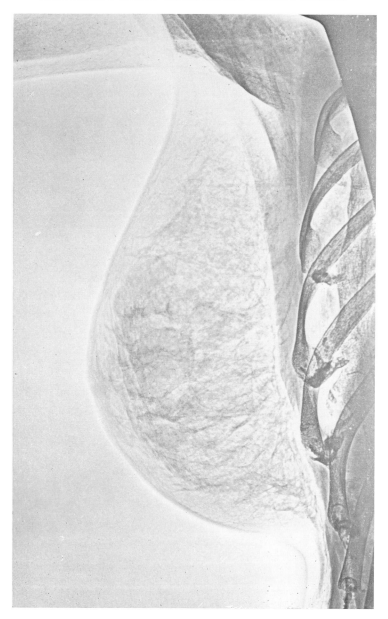

Figure 93 C *(Continued)*

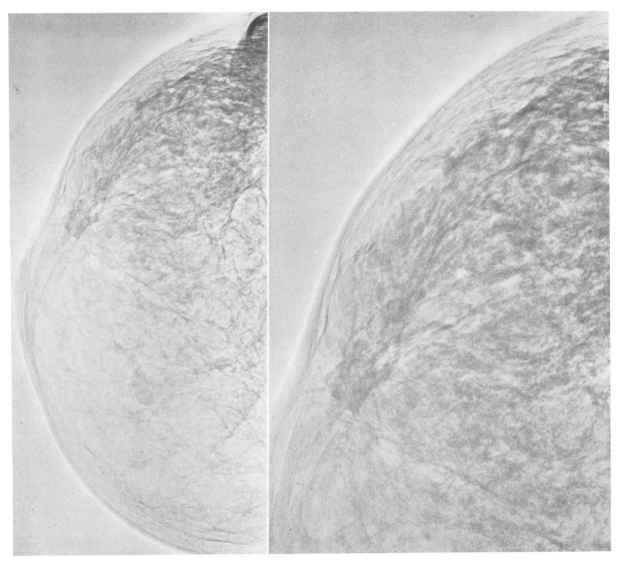

Figure 93 D-E *(Continued)*

Chapter XI

Papillomas

PAPILLOMAS ARE RARELY diagnosed correctly by plain radiographs. Occasionally a sharply contoured subareolar mass is tentatively identified as a papilloma but always with a differential diagnosis to include fibroadenoma, cyst, or even a circumscribed form of carcinoma. Most are not even visualized due to their small size and this, together with the considerable density, often within the subareolar area, precludes their identification.

They are not necessarily limited to the subareolar area. They can be seen in other parts of the breast and are, at times, multiple. Again, the correct diagnosis, especially when they are outside the subareolar area, is exceedingly difficult.

Most papillomas are not palpable. The patient may complain of a bloody nipple discharge. Those few that are palpable present as soft, freely movable tumors, and have none of the usual physical findings of malignancy. A notable exception to the concept of papillomas being small tumors in one case in which there was a subareolar mass measuring 10 centimeters in diameter. It was falsely diagnosed as a cystosarcoma. A papilloma was also present in the opposite subareolar area which tripled in size over an eight-year period. (Figs. 94, 95, 96, 97, 98, 99)

Galactography can be employed to find papillomas that are not palpable and which cannot be localized on the plain mammogram. However, at Hutzel Hospital, the surgeon is inclined to do a wedge resection of the suspected area which is localized either by palpation and/or mammography.

They sometimes calcify and when they do, they are invariably diagnosed as representing a fibroadenoma or carcinoma.

Although most papillomas that are visible on a mammogram are found in the subareolar area, it must be emphasized again that of all the subareolar tumors, papillomas are probably the *least* common. Fibroadenomas have a propensity for that location, especially in young women and girls. Some carcinomas are also seen there as discrete masses, especially in the older age group of women with fatty breasts.

One suspected papilloma which presented as a rather distinct subareolar mass 2 centimeters in diameter was found after excision to be a lobular carcinoma *in situ*. This case is unusual. First of all, because lobular carcinomas *in situ* do not appear as distinct masses. Secondly, because they are rarely found in the subareolar area or in breasts composed mainly of fat with very little dysplasia present. Lobular carcinoma *in situ* is most frequently found in breasts with considerable epithelial and connective tissue within them. (Fig. 100)

Another tumor presenting the differential diagnosis of papilloma versus some other abnormality is a medullary carcinoma with a subareolar location. According to the history, it was barely palpable and, in fact, the pathologist had some difficulty in finding it in the operative specimen. (Fig. 101)

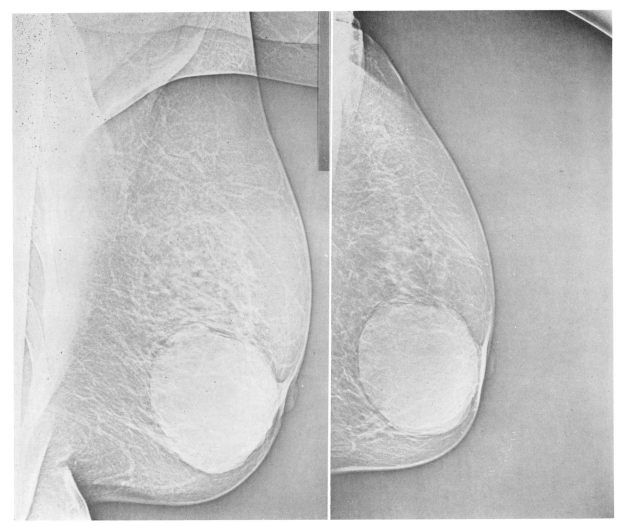

Figure 94.

HISTORY: A fifty-eight-year-old woman with a mass palpable in the subareolar area of the left breast.

RADIOGRAPHIC OBSERVATIONS: A large mass was readily observed. It was noted to have a fairly sharp margin, and in some areas there was a suggestion of compressed fat. Clear evidence of a carcinoma could not be identified.

The associated moderate involvement of the breast with a prominent duct pattern was seen.

IMPRESSION: Fibroadenoma with an outside possibility of medullary carcinoma.

HISTOPATHOLOGY: Papilloma.

DISCUSSION: This represents another unusual case of papilloma because of its large size. At the time of surgery the papilloma was noted to contain a great deal of blood and necrotic material.

This again illustrates the difficulty encountered with papillomas in arriving at the correct preoperative diagnosis. A medullary carcinoma could have an appearance exactly like this as could a cyst or fibroadenoma.

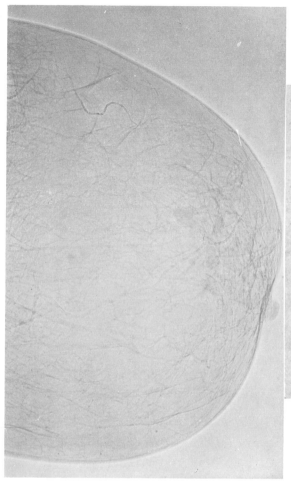

Figure 95.

HISTORY: A seventy-nine-year-old, gravida 4 woman had thickening palpable in both breasts and a clinical impression of an indeterminate nature.

RADIOGRAPHIC OBSERVATIONS: The breasts were noted to be composed mainly of fat. The main observation concerned the small mass visible in the right breast. It was noted not to have perfectly sharp margins. In addition, there were some rather large duct-like structures on the right side.

IMPRESSION: Probably a benign tumor, however, a medullary carcinoma could not be excluded.

HISTOPATHOLOGY: Papilloma.

DISCUSSION: Papillomas are exceedingly difficult to diagnose correctly and invariably if they lack calcifications, they are suspected of representing medullary carcinomas.

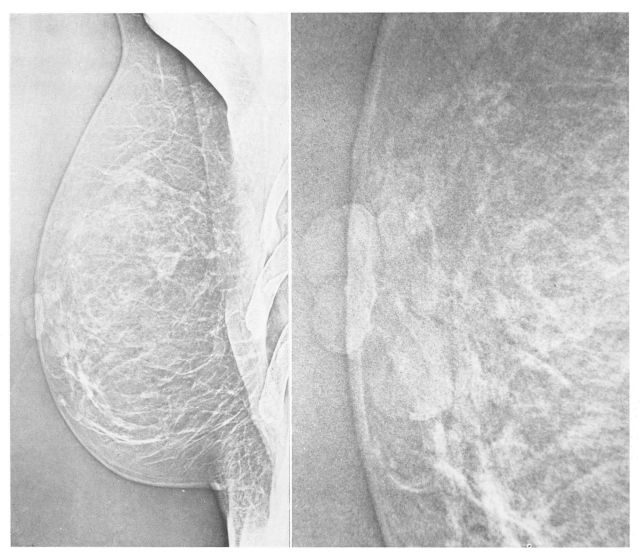

Figure 96.

HISTORY: A thirty-seven-year-old, gravida 3 woman had a mass in the subareolar area of the left breast.

RADIOGRAPHIC OBSERVATIONS: The breast was judged to be involved with minor degrees of mammary dysplasia. A distinct mass beneath the nipple was observed and it was noted to have a sharp margin without nodularity.

IMPRESSION: Probable papilloma.

HISTOPATHOLOGY: Papilloma.

DISCUSSION: The tumor has a sharp margin. The breast is involved generally with minor degrees of mammary dysplasia, and the probable site of carcinoma in this patient would be somewhere other than the subareolar area. Most important, the mass has none of the usual signs of carcinoma.

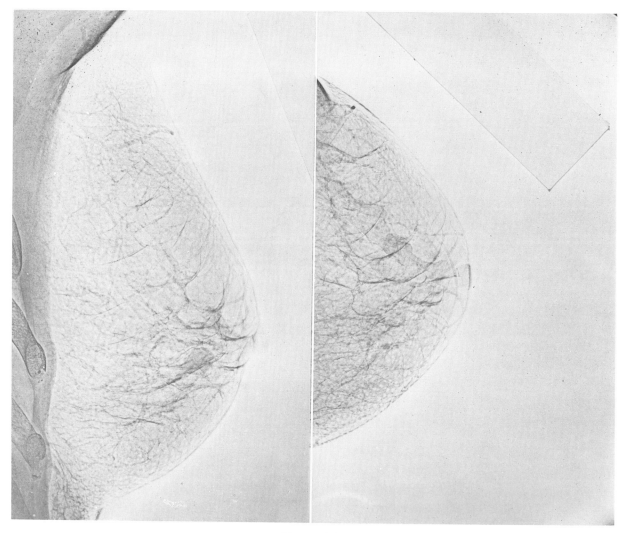

Figure 97.

HISTORY: A forty-seven-year-old, gravida 3 woman discovered a mass in her right breast. The clinical examination revealed what was thought to be a benign tumor.

RADIOGRAPHIC OBSERVATIONS: The mass in the axillary portion of the right breast was readily identified. It appeared to be associated with at least one large prominent duct extending to the subareolar area. Although the mass was fairly well circumscribed, there was really no sharp segment to its margin and for that reason it was considered with suspicion for carcinoma.

IMPRESSION: Suspicion of carcinoma with a differential diagnosis to include papilloma.

HISTOPATHOLOGY: Papilloma.

DISCUSSION: Papillomas always present problems in diagnosis. If they are seen at all, they are usually interpreted as representing carcinomas or a form of benign tumor such as fibroadenoma or cyst. When a papilloma is associated with a large dilated duct, carcinoma is always a consideration, although given the circumstances of this case, the likelihood of malignancy is probably as small as 25 percent.

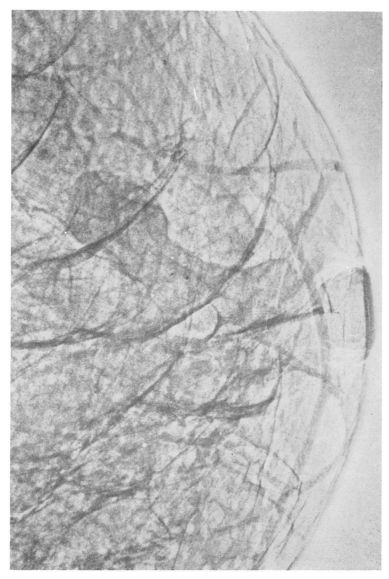

Figure 97 C *(Continued)*

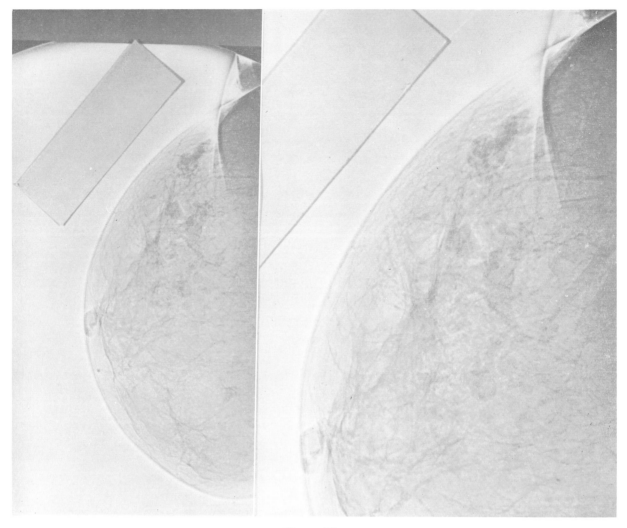

Figure 98.

HISTORY: A thirty-eight-year-old, gravida 4 woman had a mass palpable in the right breast in the upper medial quadrant.

RADIOGRAPHIC OBSERVATIONS: The mammogram of the right breast is not shown. It contained a spiculated density with numerous tumor calcifications and represented a carcinoma.

The left breast contained multiple masses in the upper axillary quadrant and they were considered unusual. They did not have the usual appearance of intramammary lymph nodes in that they were more numerous than what is usually observed. Also, they appeared "clustered."

It was not known exactly what the multiple masses represented. It was thought that perhaps they could be multiple intraductal carcinomas.

IMPRESSION: Suspicion of carcinoma, left breast. Strong impression of carcinoma, right breast (not shown).

HISTOPATHOLOGY: Intraductal papillomas, left breast; carcinoma, right breast.

DISCUSSION: This is an unusual case. First of all, most intraductal papillomas are not visualized radiographically. Secondly, when they are observed, the correct diagnosis is usually not given. Multiple papillomas as seen in this case are a rare occurrence.

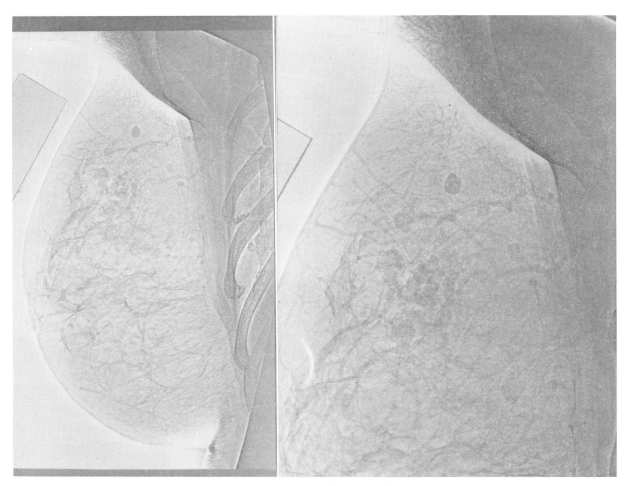

Figure 98 C-D *(Continued)*

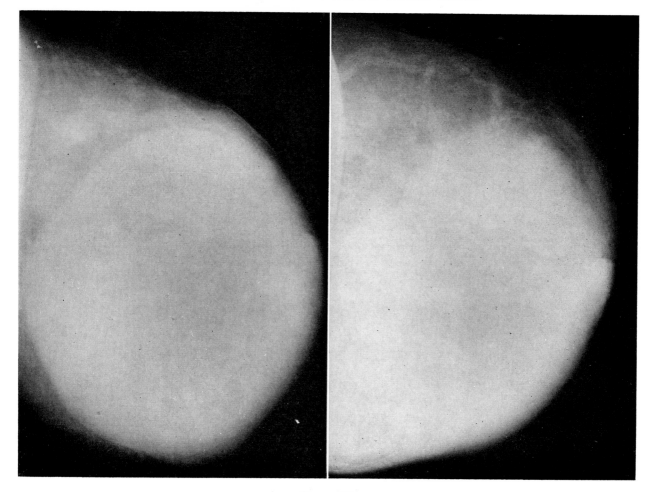

Figure 99.

HISTORY: A sixty-year-old woman had a very large mass palpable in her breast and a clinical impression of carcinoma. The patient had congestive heart failure.

RADIOGRAPHIC OBSERVATIONS: The huge mass in the subareolar area was readily identified. In one projection it was noted to have a rather sharp margin. No calcifications were associated with it.

IMPRESSION: Cystosarcoma phylloides with a differential diagnosis to include giant fibroadenoma or other forms of sarcoma.

HISTOPATHOLOGY: Papilloma with necrosis.

DISCUSSION: This is an extremely large papilloma, measuring 10 cms in diameter on the original image. Certainly one would have great difficulty in arriving at the correct diagnosis.

The case is interesting in that, because of the woman's heart disease, she was not operated on for a considerable period of time. There was bleeding into the tumor and necrosis which eventually erupted through the skin to become infected with a gas-producing organism.

She had a large papilloma measuring 4 cms in diameter in the opposite subareolar area.

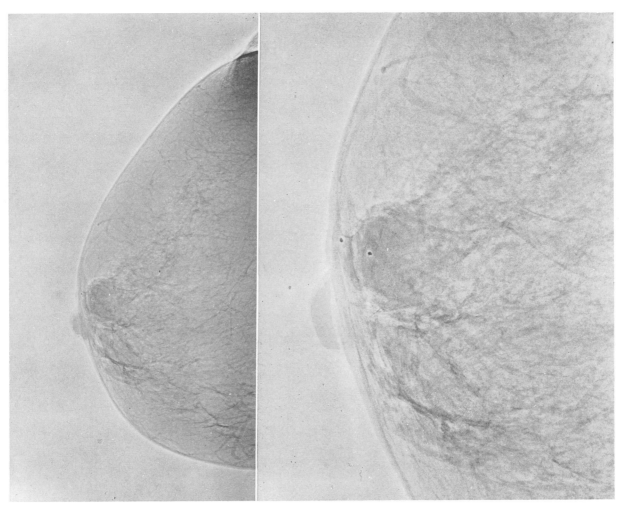

Figure 100.

HISTORY: A fifty-five-year-old, gravida 2 woman discovered a mass beneath the nipple apparently of two weeks duration. Physical examination was not remarkable and the clinical impression was benign disease.

RADIOGRAPHIC OBSERVATIONS: The mass-like density in the subareolar area could be identified rather readily. At no point was it sharply circumscribed. The calcifications were considered unrelated.

IMPRESSION: Suspicion of carcinoma with a differential diagnosis of papilloma.

HISTOPATHOLOGY: Lobular carcinoma.

DISCUSSION: A mass of this type proves to be malignant only about 20 to 25 percent of the time. At the time of operation it appeared to represent a papilloma, but on the permanent sections it was judged to be a lobular carcinoma. The subareolar location is unusual for lobular carcinoma, they are more commonly seen in the depths of the breast and accompanied by dysplasia.

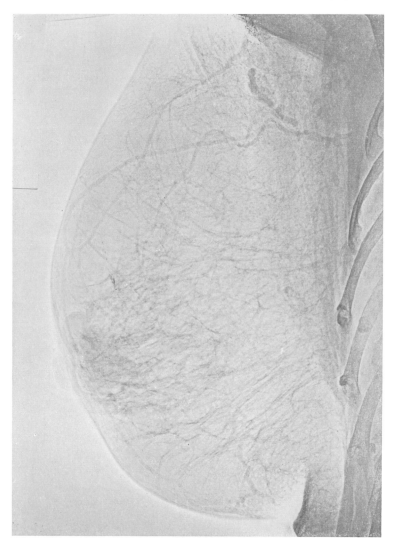

Figure 100 C *(Continued)*

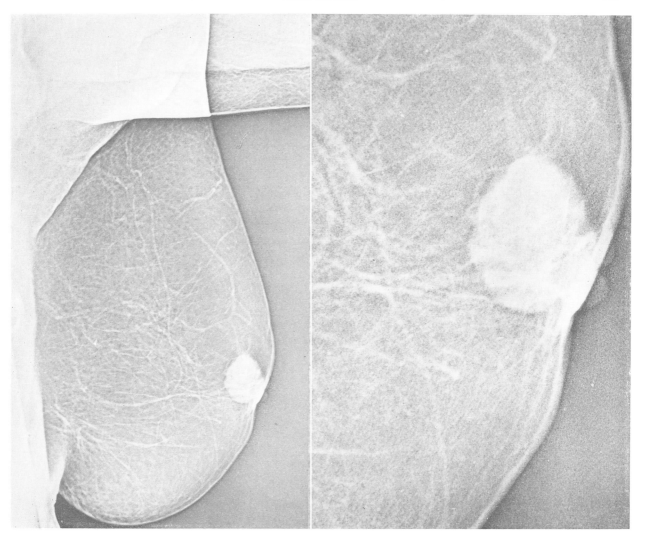

Figure 101.

HISTORY: A seventy-four-year-old, nulliparous woman had a mass in the right breast near the nipple, of six month's duration and a clinical impression of benign disease.

RADIOGRAPHIC OBSERVATIONS: A very distinct mass in the subareolar area of the breast was the chief observation. It was noted to have a somewhat finely nodular margin. The breast was composed mainly of fat. In the opposite breast (not shown) was a 1 cm mass containing aggregates of calcification, and that was interpreted as being a fibroadenoma which was correct.

IMPRESSION: Carcinoma, right breast, probably medullary.

HISTOPATHOLOGY: Carcinoma, medullary.

DISCUSSION: The very anterior location of the carcinoma is not surprising in that there is no active glandular tissue seen in the other portions of the breast.

This tumor differs from the usual papilloma in that it has a distinctly nodular margin, whereas the few papillomas which have been diagnosed correctly have had a very sharp margin. The tumor was barely palpable to the surgeon and even to the pathologist. This is not surprising as medullary carcinomas tend to be "soft."

Chapter XII

Fat Necrosis

Fᴀᴛ ɴᴇᴄʀᴏsɪs ɪs ᴜsᴜᴀʟʟʏ associated with trauma, either from a direct blow or from a biopsy. It has a rather characteristic early appearance, especially when associated with biopsy. Seen early, there are sharply circumscribed areas of lessened density at the operative site which later tend to calcify in a characteristic eggshell form. Later they present as less perfect, densely calcified spheres or ovals. Very infrequently the area of fat necrosis presents as a solid tumor which may be irregular or nodular making it difficult to exclude the possibility of malignancy. (Figs. 102, 103)

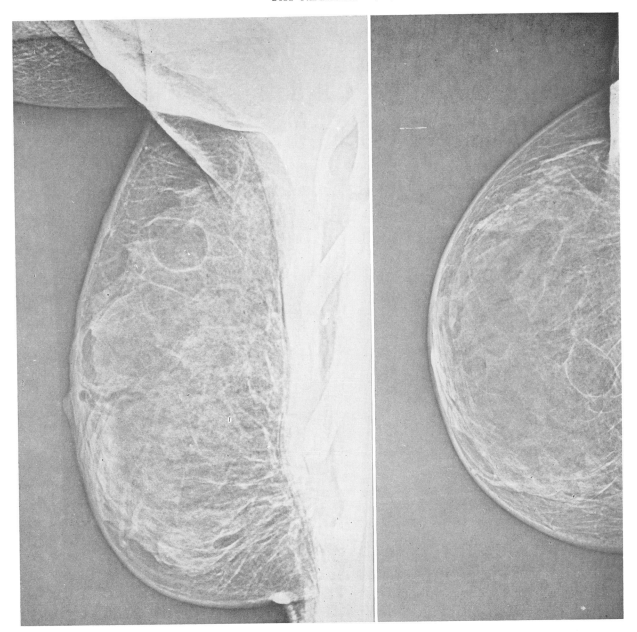

Figure 102.

HISTORY: A thirty-one-year-old, gravida 2 woman had a biopsy of the breast approximately five months before this examination.

RADIOGRAPHIC OBSERVATIONS: The breasts were noted to be involved severely with mammary dysplasia. The chief interest was the mass in the upper quadrant which was noted to have a fat density and very sharp margination. Associated with it was slight thickening of the skin, seen on the lateral projection, at the site of the biopsy.

IMPRESSION: Fat necrosis from previous biopsy.

HISTOPATHOLOGY: None.

DISCUSSION: It is unusual to see areas of fat necrosis from biopsy as large as in this particular case. Very frequently they are not more than a centimeter in diameter and are usually multiple.

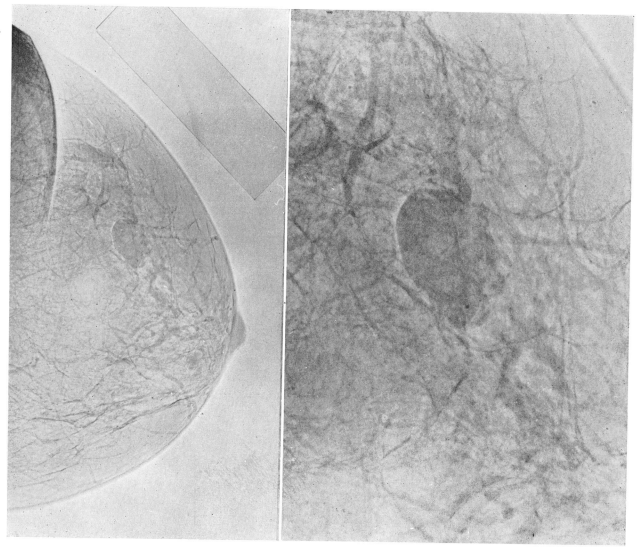

Figure 103.

HISTORY: A forty-three-year-old, gravida 5 woman came for a routine examination of the breasts.

RADIOGRAPHIC OBSERVATIONS: The breasts were noted to be composed mainly of fat with a few prominent ducts in the subareolar area. A mass in the axillary portion was identified and its margin, for the most part, appeared to be very sharp and distinct with slight lobularity anteriorly. No clear area of invasion as from a malignancy could be identified.

IMPRESSION: Fibroadenoma with an outside possibility of medullary carcinoma and a recommendation that if the tumor was not excised, the patient should be followed very carefully.

HISTOPATHOLOGY: Fat necrosis.

DISCUSSION: Because the mass is lobular in one area and sharply bounded in another, the most likely diagnosis is fibroadenoma. Medullary carcinomas often have an identical form and cannot be excluded from consideration. Surprisingly, this tumor represents an area of fat necrosis. Fat necrosis associated with previous biopsy and hematoma usually presents as areas of lucency, very sharply circumscribed, round or oval in configuration. Eventually such areas will calcify.

Chapter XIII

Lipomas

LIPOMAS ARE DISCRETE, noncalcified breast masses. They pose no problem in diagnosis due to the lessened absorption coefficient of the contents, and they present on the mammogram as an area of lessened density. In the fatty breast, however, lipomas are difficult to identify, and identification is done mainly by visualizing the very thin capsule.

The usual history is that of a palpable mass within the breast of long duration. It should be stated, however, that most are not palpable and are discovered only accidentally by mammography when it is done for some other reason.

The radiographic features are those of a mass frequently lobulated and faintly encapsulated. If the lipoma occurs in a dense breast with a great deal of dysplasia, it is readily visible. If, however, it is in a fatty breast, it can be very difficult to see. They are rarely seen in men. (Figs. 104, 105)

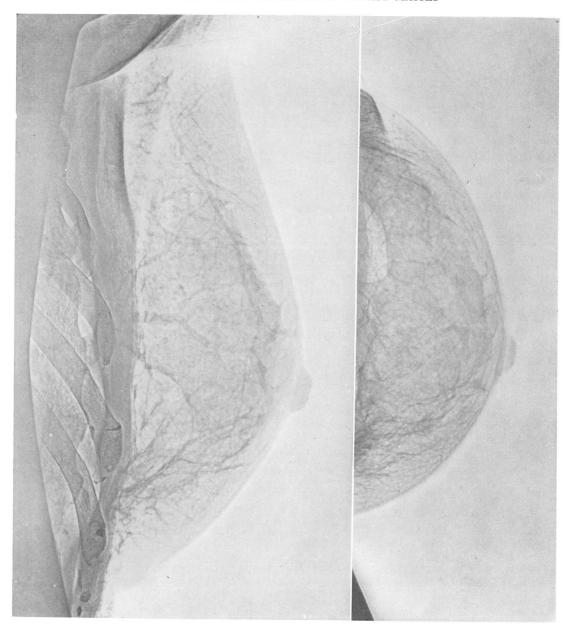

Figure 104.

HISTORY: A forty-eight-year-old, gravida 4 woman discovered a mass in her right breast. The clinical impression was benign disease.

RADIOGRAPHIC OBSERVATIONS: The breasts were noted to be involved rather severely with dysplasia. The radiolucent, sharply circumscribed mass in the lower axillary quadrant of the breast was considered very characteristic for lipoma.

IMPRESSION: Lipoma.

HISTOPATHOLOGY: None.

DISCUSSION: The patient has been seen over an eight-year period and there has not been a change in the tumor. A very confident impression of lipoma can be made because of the relative lucency and sharp circumscription of the tumor.

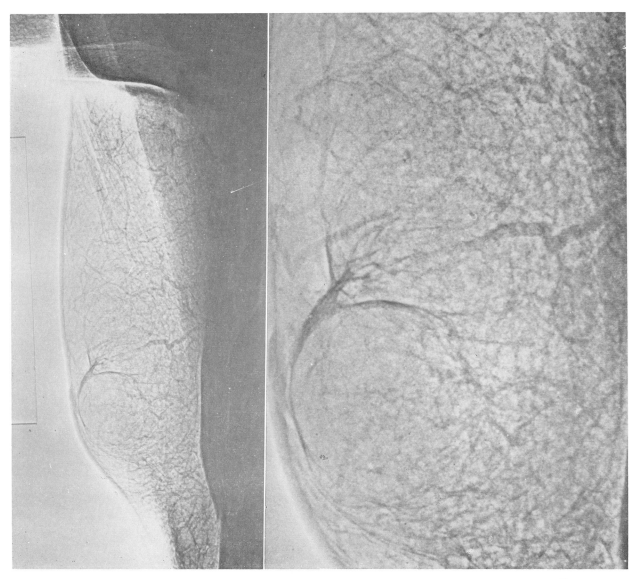

Figure 105.

HISTORY: A sixty-one-year-old man had a palpable mass in the left breast and a clinical impression of benign disease.

RADIOGRAPHIC OBSERVATIONS: The breast appeared to be composed mainly of fat and uninvolved with gynecomastia. The very faint encapsulated area of radiolucency beneath the nipple and areola was noted and it was concluded that it was composed of fat.

IMPRESSION: Lipoma, left breast.

HISTOPATHOLOGY: Lipoma.

DISCUSSION: It is difficult to identify lipomas in breasts composed mainly of fat. One sees them best by virtue of their encapsulation rather than by virtue of a difference in density. On the other hand, if the breast is dense, they are observed most often as areas of relative radiolucency.

Chapter XIV

Galactoceles

GALACTOCELES are interesting. They appear as small, fatty tumors which are rarely seen on mammography. When seen, they are most frequently in the dense breast where the sharp contrast between the fat content of the galactocele and the surrounding dysplasia is very striking. They are accidental observations and are not palpable.

Radiographically they are very sharply limited, usually 1.0 to 1.5 centimeters in diameter, round, or more frequently, ovoid in configuration. They are typically multiple and very often bilateral. Galactoceles are merely another manifestation of retained lactiferous material within ducts. The duct becomes obstructed and dilated. (Figs. 106, 107, 108, 109)

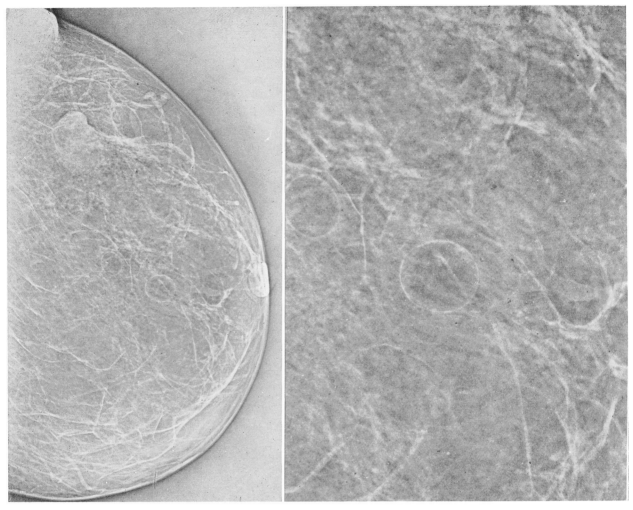

Figure 106.

HISTORY: A twenty-five-year-old, gravida 2 woman had a biopsy of the right breast eight months before this examination and now has a mass palpable in the right breast.

RADIOGRAPHIC OBSERVATIONS: The mass in the axillary quadrant was identified readily and noted to have irregular medial and anterior margins.

The three very sharp circumscribed areas of radiolucency in the central portion of the breast were also observed.

IMPRESSION: Galactocele, probable fibroadenoma (see discussion, Fig. 43).

HISTOPATHOLOGY: Fibroadenoma and galactocele.

DISCUSSION: Galactoceles are very infrequently observed and the appearance here is considered very characteristic. The area of lucency should be small, round or oval in form and extremely sharply circumscribed.

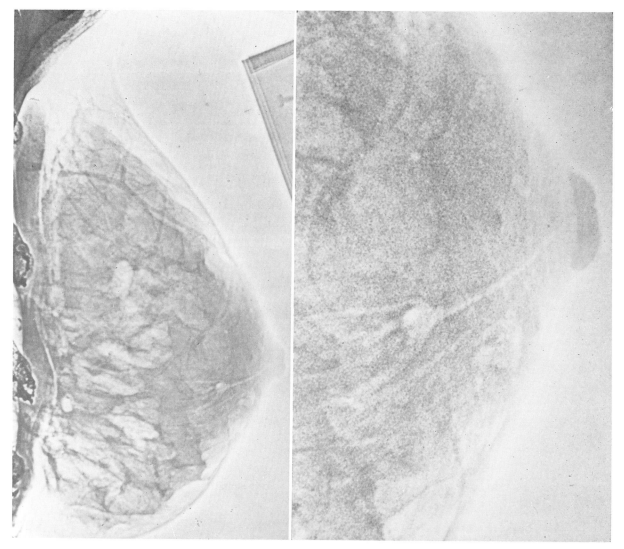

Figure 107.

HISTORY: A thirty-five-year-old, gravida 3 woman whose last pregnancy was seven years before this examination. She had thickening palpable in both breasts and a clinical impression of benign disease.

RADIOGRAPHIC OBSERVATIONS: The breasts were noted to be somewhat dense and involved with dysplasia. The interesting observation concerned the somewhat linear and rounded areas of diminished density located in the subareolar regions. Because of their lessened opacity, they were thought to be composed of fat.

IMPRESSION: Retained lactiferous material in terminal ducts with cystic dilatation.

HISTOPATHOLOGY: None.

DISCUSSION: Retained lactiferous material is an interesting and fairly common observation but it has little known significance. It is identified most readily if the subareolar area is quite dense. It may occur years after pregnancy and has been observed in nulliparous women. Often it is accompanied by cystic dilatations producing small mass-like areas of lessened density which should not be confused with lipomas or galactoceles.

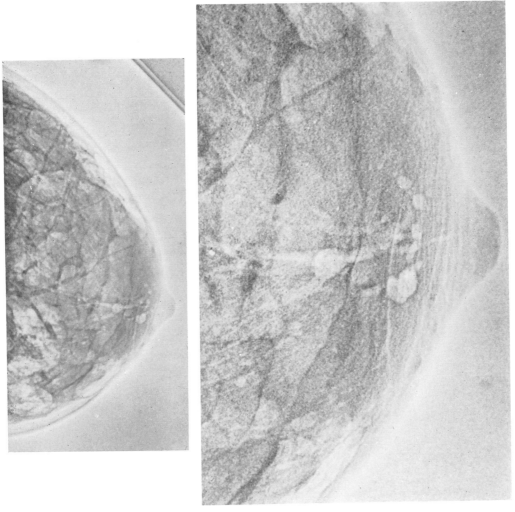

Figure 107 C-D *(Continued)*

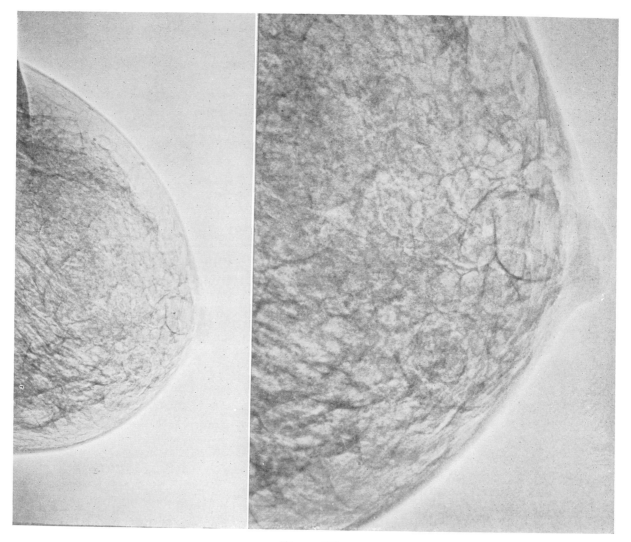

Figure 108.

HISTORY: A thirty-nine-year-old, gravida 3 woman had masses palpable in both breasts and a clinical impression of cystic disease.

RADIOGRAPHIC OBSERVATIONS: The general density of the breast was felt consistent with mammary dysplasia—a combination of cystic disease and adenosis. The interesting observations concerned the areas, rather sharply circumscribed, in the subareolar regions bilaterally.

IMPRESSION: Retained lactiferous material with cystic dilatation of terminal ducts.

HISTOPATHOLOGY: None.

DISCUSSION: It is very common to observe retained lactiferous material in ducts. Usually it has a linear pattern. At times it forms circumscribed patterns, as seen here.

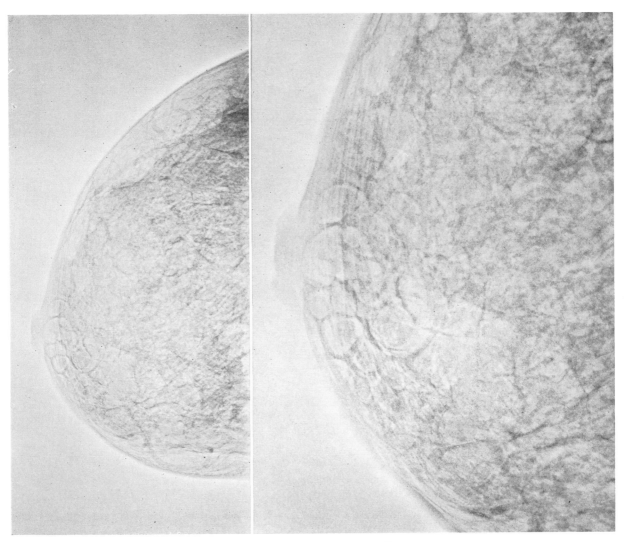

Figure 108 C-D *(Continued)*

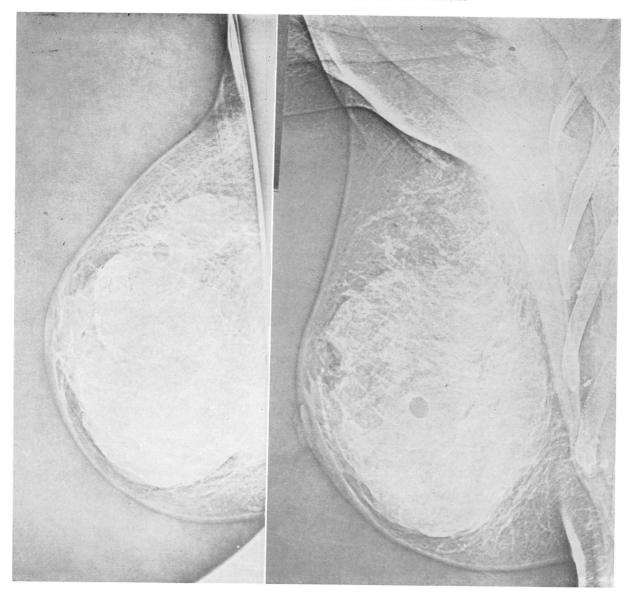

Figure 109.

HISTORY: A forty-five-year-old, gravida 2 woman has palpable abnormalities in both breasts. Her physican thought there was a dominant mass on the left side, and he attempted but failed to aspirate it.

RADIOGRAPHIC OBSERVATIONS: The examination was made two days after the attempted aspiration. The sharply circumscribed area of lucency was considered to represent an air bubble introduced at the time of attempted aspiration.

IMPRESSION: Air bubble from attempted aspiration.

HISTOPATHOLOGY: None.

DISCUSSION: The small lucent area simulates a galactocele although galactoceles are frequently multiple. It should not be confused with a small lipoma because lipomas tend to be lobulated, and they are not as sharply circumscribed.

Chapter XV

Skin and Subcutaneous Area

ABNORMALITIES OF THE SKIN and subcutaneous area pose no problem in diagnosis when the X-ray beam happens to catch them tangentially. When this fortuitous positioning does not occur, they will project as though they were within the breast. This potential error exists in the instance of masses and also in diseases of the skin causing calcifications.

The history of the patient is usually not significant for the particular skin abnormality. Because it probably has been present for a long period of time and because the patient is usually being examined for an abnormality within the breast, she will often fail to mention the skin abnormality.

The technologist should look at the skin of the breast very carefully and note any abnormality and if there is any question as to its nature from the radiographic point of view, additional views should be made with the skin abnormality tangential to the X-ray beam.

Radiographically, they usually present as sharply circumscribed tumors. There are many types, the most common of which are nevi and epithelial inclusion or sebaceous cysts. More exotic forms such as keloids, Van Recklinghausen's disease, and primary skin neoplasms are rarely seen. (Figs. 110, 111, 112, 113)

Another form of skin pathology occasionally encountered is xanthoma of the skin. These tumors are characterized by fatty deposits and present as lucent areas on the mammogram and pose no problem in diagnosis. They are usually multiple and bilateral. In some areas, one of the small tumors will be imaged tangentially, and their cutaneous location will become very apparent.

Probably the most important aspects of this section on the skin are first, that the radiologist should be constantly on the alert for the possible errors that may occur as a result of skin abnormalities. Secondly, that the technologists should be instructed to pay particular attention to abnormalities of the skin and map them on a diagram for the radiologist's use at the time of interpretation. This is even more important when the skin abnormality is characterized only by calcifications. Always to be considered is the fact that the skin abnormality will present very frequently on both views of the breast as though it is within the interior of the breast. Without having tangential views or precise information from the technologist, it is impossible to make a reasonable diagnosis.

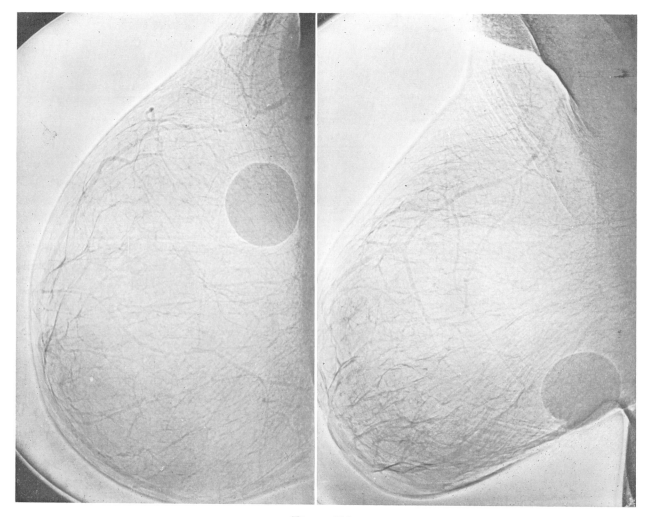

Figure 110.

HISTORY: A fifty-year-old, nulliparous woman discovered a lump in the lower lateral quadrant of the left breast. The clinical impression was benign disease.

RADIOGRAPHIC OBSERVATIONS: The breasts were noted to be composed chiefly of fat and essentially normal. A very sharply circumscribed, subcutaneous tumor was observed, measuring about 3 cms in diameter.

IMPRESSION: Epithelial inclusion cyst.

HISTOPATHOLOGY: Epithelial inclusion cyst.

DISCUSSION: The very sharp limitation of the tumor, together with the subcutaneous location, should lead one to the correct impression.

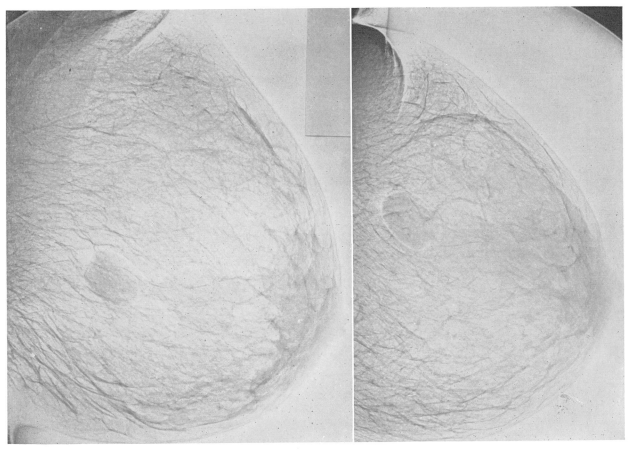

Figure 111.

HISTORY: A twenty-one-year-old, gravida 2 woman has had a mass on the skin of the right breast for approximately one year which recently has enlarged. The clinical impression was keloid.

RADIOGRAPHIC OBSERVATIONS: When one considered the routine caudal and lateral projections of the breast, the mass was placed within the parenchyma of the breast and one would be inclined to identify it as a benign tumor, most likely a fibroadenoma. The tangential view, however, showed clearly that it arose from the skin.

IMPRESSION: Keloid with other types of skin tumors included in the differential diagnosis.

HISTOPATHOLOGY: Dermatofibrosarcoma protuberans of the skin.

DISCUSSION: This tumor occurs rarely. It will recur locally and has been known to metastasize if not widely excised. It is important to note that skin tumors may appear to be intramammary if seen on only two projections. The additional tangential view that shows the origin of the tumor is essential to correct diagnosis.

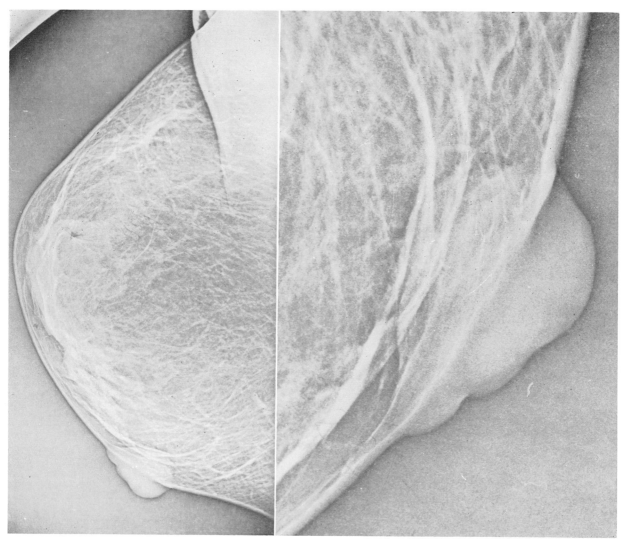

Figure 111 C-D *(Continued)*

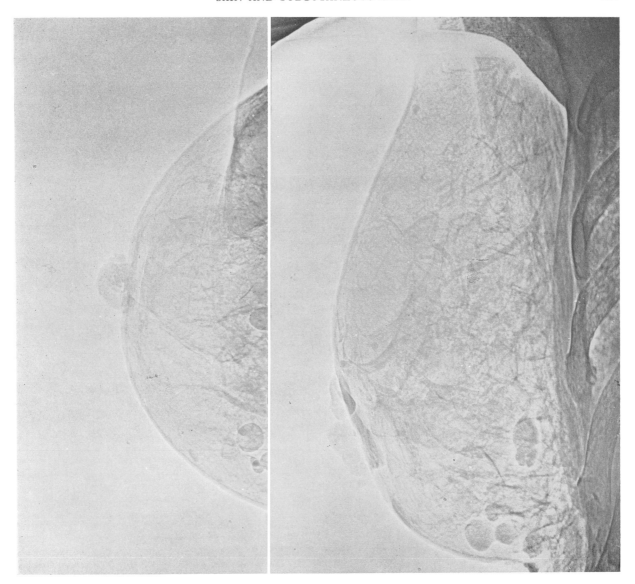

Figure 112.

HISTORY: A fifty-one-year-old, gravida 3 woman with a family history of breast cancer and thickening palpable in the left breast. She had a right mastectomy five years before this examination.

RADIOGRAPHIC OBSERVATIONS: The breasts were noted to be involved with mammary dysplasia. The interesting aspect of the study was the multiple cutaneous tumors which were noted to be well circumscribed.

IMPRESSION: Von Recklinghausen's disease.

HISTOPATHOLOGY: None.

DISCUSSION: The interpretation is considered straightforward. The multiplicity of the tumors plus the fact that some are seen tangentially to the skin, makes the diagnosis easy.

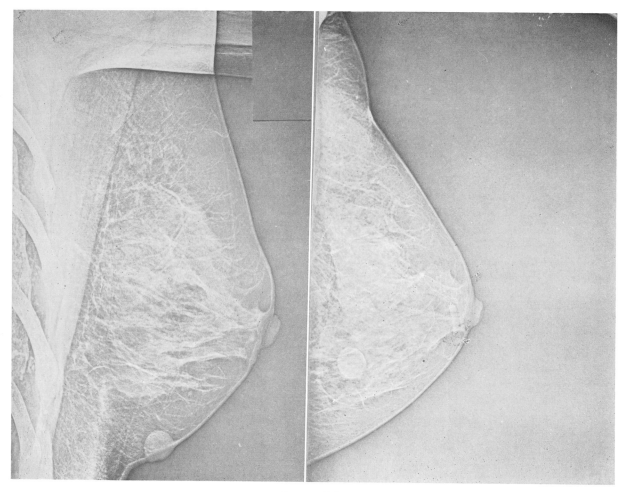

Figure 113.

HISTORY: A thirty-seven-year-old, gravida 4 woman had thickening palpable in both breasts and a clinical impression of benign disease.

RADIOGRAPHIC OBSERVATIONS: The breasts were involved rather symmetrically with minor degrees of mammary dysplasia. The interesting aspect of the case was the tumor arising from the skin of the breast which just happened to be caught tangentially in the routine lateral view.

IMPRESSION: Skin tumor, probably epidermal inclusion cyst or sebaceous cyst.

HISTOPATHOLOGY: None.

DISCUSSION: The placement of the tumor in the cutaneous region is simple in this particular case because the lateral projection happens to be optimum for imaging the mass tangentially.

Chapter XVI

Differential Diagnosis: Benign versus Malignant

THE PRIMARY PURPOSE of this section is to make the radiologist aware of the features that distinguish benign from malignant, discrete masses which do not have calcifications. Identification of the type of benign mass is secondary. The carcinoma which presents as a problem is nearly always a medullary one. It is a difficult differential diagnosis, and one must employ the history and physical findings, radiographic appearance, and consider what is likely to be present in a given set of circumstances. In coming to any opinion, the following guidelines may be used:

DIFFERENTIAL DIAGNOSIS

HISTORICAL	MALIGNANT	BENIGN
Age	Infrequent under the age of 30	Any age but very common under the age of 30
Pain	Frequent	Frequent in the instance of cysts
Nonsanguinous nipple discharge	No value	No value
Sanguinous nipple discharge	Important especially if there are associated large discrete ducts	No correlation except in papilloma
Aspirable	Very rare (carcinoma arising in cyst)	The usual features of cysts
Rapidity of appearance	No value	No value, although a frequent observation by the patient in cases of cyst
Rapid diminution in size	Great value and speaks against malignancy	Great value. Very characteristic for cysts
Rapid enlargement (days or few weeks)	Usually against malignancy, possible exception is sarcoma.	Great value. Very characteristic for cysts

PHYSICAL EXAMINATION

Palpability	No value. Some large medullary carcinomas are nonpalpable.	No value
Not fixed	No value	No value
Cystic consistency	No value. Typical for cystosarcoma phylloides	No value

Skin retraction	Not characteristic for the well-circumscribed carcinoma. Seen often in the spiculated variety.	Fat necrosis will rarely exhibit retraction.
Skin and/or areolar edema	Present only in advanced cases	Very common in acute abscess
Palpable axillary nodes	Valuable sign	Commonly observed in abscess
Increased superficial venous vascularity	Occurs in some sarcomas	No association

RADIOGRAPHIC

Number	Unusual to be multiple (coexistence of benign with malignant is not uncommon)	Very common to be multiple
Bilaterality	Uncommon	Extremely common
Location	Limited value. Tend to be "within" active breast tissue	Limited value. The vast majority of "superficially placed" tumors are benign.
Subareolar location	No value	No value
Sharp contour	Limited value. Occasionally seen.	Characteristic of cyst and other types.
Lobulated contour	Limited value. Occasionally seen.	Characteristic of fibro-adenomas.
Nodular contour	Forces diagnosis of malignancy but often will lead to false-positive diagnosis.	Occurs not infrequently in fibroadenomas.
Tapered contour	Forces diagnosis of malignancy but often will lead to false-positive diagnosis.	Occurs frequently in cyst and fibroadenomas.
Environment: fat	Of value. Relatively uncommon for carcinomas.	Common, especially in fibro-adenomas, lymph nodes and other benign tumors.
Environment: dysplasia	Significant value, especially in older age group	No value
Environment: prominent duct pattern	Significant value	No value
Change in size on interval examination at 3 months: enlargement	Unusual to observe significant change except in sarcomas	Significant enlargement in size of cysts is common.
Change in size on interval examination at 3 months: reduction	Does not occur	Common in cysts, abscess and hematoma.
Change in contour on interval examination at 3 months	Wall becomes obviously nodular or irregular	Cysts may have a more irregular contour if they decrease in size.

All things must be considered in unison, but a few remarks will be made about each of the points from the list.

Age of Patient

Age plays a dominant role in influencing the final radiographic opinion. It is sufficiently important in the consideration of all solitary, palpable, freely movable masses in women under the age of thirty. One could diagnose fibroadenoma on the basis of the history features alone and be right 95 percent of the time. As we consider older women, a carcinoma becomes more and more likely; but the significant majority of uncalcified discrete breast masses in women between the ages of sixty and seventy are benign tumors.

Pain

Pain is not a good differentiating historical feature. It is not uncommon for carcinomas to be accompanied by pain, nor is this complaint uncommon in the instance of cysts. Pain, of course, is the routine complaint in women with breast abscesses.

Nipple Discharge

A nonsanguinous nipple discharge is of no value in differentiating between benign and malignant breast masses and is considered coincidental.

A sanguinous nipple discharge is important in the diagnosis of malignancies. It is most often seen in cases of comedocarcinoma, which are often accompanied by calcifications. When one is dealing with a rather discrete mass representing a carcinoma and there is a sanguinous nipple discharge, it is usually an intraductal carcinoma and the physician can often identify one or several rather large discrete ducts associated with it. Insofar as the benign conditions are concerned, there is no correlation except in the cases of papilloma where there is frequently a history of such a discharge.

Aspiration

Aspiration is a good diagnostic and therapeutic procedure which should be encouraged. It should be done only when there is a preponderance of evidence toward a benign cyst, both from the mammographic appearance and physical findings. Failing to aspirate a mass necessitates that either the patient be followed by repeat physical and radiographic examination or that the tumor be excised.

Rapidity of Appearance

This feature of the history is of limited value. It is probably an accurate observation in cystic disease when the patient states that the mass seemed to appear "overnight." It cannot be relied upon too heavily, however, because very often it is related merely to discovery. That is to say, the mass had gone unobserved until suddenly the patient became aware of it by one means or another.

Change in Size

A rapid diminution in size of the palpable mass is of great value in the diagnosis of cysts. It is not at all unusual for the patient to discover a mass suddenly, visit her physician, and then after several more days appear for the radiographic examination only to state that the mass is no longer present. The diminution in size or disappearance, of course, speaks against malignancy, but there must be some caution used in the evaluation of this observation by the patient. The mass may be a small tumor that is palpable in one position but not in others.

Very rapid enlargement of a mass is of considerable diagnostic value in that it is often observed in the instance of cysts. Other benign tumors do not enlarge rapidly. Carcinomas do not usually increase in size in a time span of only a few weeks although sarcomas may.

Palpability

The fact that a particular well-circumscribed, uncalcified mass is or is not palpable is not of great value in distinguishing between benign and malignant disease. Medullary carcinomas are notable for being rather soft with no desmoplastic reaction and, for that reason, can be quite large and still nonpalpable. Benign tumors, on the other hand, are very readily palpable. It is likely the 1 centimeter fibroadenoma or cyst can be palpated more frequently than the 1 centimeter medullary carcinoma.

Fixation

This is not considered to be of value. As a matter of fact, fat necrosis is more likely to feel "fixed" than is the typical medullary carcinoma.

Consistency

This is not considered of value. Medullary carcinomas, being somewhat soft, can have a cystic feel and, of course, cystosarcoma phylloides is characterized as having a cystic consistency.

Skin Changes

Skin retraction is not characteristic of the well-circumscribed carcinoma. It is very often seen in carcinomas of the spiculated variety. The only benign condition which may produce skin retraction, as one considers discrete masses, is fat necrosis.

Skin and/or areolar edema is not seen often in the carcinomas characterized as discrete masses and when it is observed, it is indicative of advanced disease. The changes are commonly observed in acute abscess.

Axillary Lymphadenopathy

This is a valuable sign in the diagnosis of carcinoma, but it is usually indicative of advanced disease. As a rule, there is no problem in arriving at the correct diagnosis merely on the basis of the observations concerning the mass itself. Acute inflammatory diseases could also produce axillary lymphadenopathy.

Increased Vascularity

This is not considered a good sign in differentiating between benign and malignant disease. Characteristically sarcomas will have a very definite increased venous vascularity.

Number

A solitary, unilateral mass is more suspect of representing a carcinoma than are multiple or bilateral masses, however. Carcinomas which present as multiple, discrete, uncalcified breast masses are rarely encountered. However, even single masses are much more apt to be benign tumors than malignant ones. The coexistence of benign masses and a malignant one is not at all uncommon. One must regard each mass separately.

Bilateral simultaneous carcinomas in the form of sharply circumscribed discrete masses have never been observed in the series of cases at Hutzel Hospital. Unilateral benign and contralateral malignant masses, however, are not uncommon. Bilateral benign tumors are extremely common, especially as one regards the intramammary lymph nodes, fibroadenomas and cysts.

Location

The factor of location has limited value. However, carcinomas tend to be "within the active part of the breast tissue," that is to say, within areas of increased density representing mammary dysplasia. Benign tumors also are likely to occur in the same area, but the benign tumors have a greater propensity to be superficially placed than do malignant ones. The subareolar location of tumors as a point in differential diagnosis is of no value. They may be benign or malignant.

Contour

Observation of contour is of value in differential diagnosis. A discrete mass with an extremely sharp contour is much more likely to be benign than malignant. However, one must keep in mind that very sharply contoured tumors are rarely carcinomas.

A lobulated contour is not a conclusive indicator. Medullary carcinomas are occasionally seen which are indistinguishable from fibroadenomas insofar as the contour is concerned. Lobulation is, of course, characteristic for fibroadenomas.

A nodular contour is of significance, although it is often misleading. It forces a diagnosis of malignancy that is frequently correct, but at the same time many fibroadenomas and some other masses within the breast will have a nodular contour.

Tapering of the ends of the mass is occasionally a feature of carcinoma, but only about 50 percent of tumors with well-tapered ends are likely to prove malignant. The other 50 percent will be benign lesions, notably cysts or fibroadenomas.

Environment

The general condition of the breast is felt to be of value in differential diagnosis. If the breast is composed almost solely of fat with very little active glandular tissue, then a sharply circumscribed mass is almost always a benign tumor. It is uncommon for a fatty breast to harbor a carcinoma. One must not forget, however, that it does occur and in the proper situation, such as the right age group, sharply circumscribed masses in a fatty breast should not be dismissed completely and at least follow-up examination obtained.

There is a significant association between severe dysplasia and carcinoma. Therefore, this environmental change has value in the differential diagnosis, especially in the women above the age of thirty-five or forty. This is considered to be the type of breast at highest risk for breast cancer. Great care should be taken in dismissing a discrete breast mass as benign in the face of significant dysplasia. Cysts, of course, are frequently observed in the dysplastic breast.

The prominent duct pattern has precisely the same relationship. Most carcinomas are accompanied by some degree of prominent duct pattern and the majority have it to a moderate or severe degree.

Fluctuation

The observation of mass enlargement on a three-month interval examination is very significant. If the enlargement is great, that is to say, if the mass increases in size by doubling or tripling, it is more characteristic of benign disease, such as a cyst, than anything else. Circumscribed carcinomas do not grow rapidly. Sarcomas may do so.

Cysts, abscesses and hematomas are commonly observed to reduce in size. Carcinomas are not. Care must be taken to keep the geometry of the comparison examination the same.

A change in the contour of a mass is exceedingly important. The carcinomas tend to become more obviously malignant, that is to say, the wall will become more nodular, irregular or spiculations may appear. In circumscribed carcinomas, this change is usually more prominent than the enlargement of the mass. Fibroadenomas change very little and their contour remains the same. Papillomas, although uncommonly observed, maintain their contours as they enlarge. Cysts will have a change in appearance of contour if they decrease in size in that they tend to look more irregular.

Dysplasia above and below a mass may obscure portions of its margin. The two projections (or more) in which the breast is always examined prevents this from occurring too frequently. However, even with multiple projections, there are many cases in which the margins simply cannot be evaluated completely. It is in cases such as these that all of the less specific indications of benign and malignant disease come into play, or that the radiologist must simply state that a confident diagnosis of either benign or malignant disease cannot be made. His recommendation might be to attempt aspiration if a cyst is suspected, or biopsy, either by needle or excision. Repeat physical examination and follow-up radiographic examinations are also of value. The actions on such difficult cases are influenced by the philosophy of the referring physician and often by the patient and the patient's own attitude toward breast biopsy or follow-up examinations.

In summary, all sources of information are utilized in trying to arrive at a correct diagnosis when confronted with a discrete uncalcified breast mass. However, one must not lose sight of the fact that if there is a question of malignancy, the report should not be worded in a manner that would discourage the referring physician from utilizing his own judgment and findings based on the physical examination and questioning of the patient.

Bibliography

1. Baclesse, F., and Willemin, A.: *Atlas of Mammography*. Paris, Librairie des Facultes, 1967.
2. Egan, R. L.: *Mammography*. Springfield, Thomas, 1964.
3. Egan, R. L.: Experience with mammography in a tumor institution. *Radiology, 6*:894-900, 1960.
4. Frankl, G., and Rosenfeld, D. D.: Breast xeroradiography: an analysis of our first 17 months. *Ann Surg, 178*:676-679, 1973.
5. Gershon-Cohen, J., and Ingleby, H.: Roentgen screening of mammary tumor progression. *Am J Roentgenol, 77*:131-137, 1957.
6. Gros, C. M.: *Diseases of the Breast*. Paris, Masson, 1963. (In French)
7. Hoeffken, W., and Lanyi, M.: *Roentgenuntersuchung der Brust; Technik, Diagnostik, Differentialdiagnose, Ergebnisse*. Stuttgart, Thieme, 1973. (In German)
8. Hyman, L. J., and Abellera, R. M.: Carcinomatous lymph nodes within breast parenchyma. *Arch Surg, 109*:759-761, 1974.
9. Ingleby, H., and Gershon-Cohen, J.: *Comparative Anatomy, Pathology and Roentgenology of the Breast*. Philadelphia, University of Pennsylvania, 1960.
10. Leborgne, R. A.: *The Breast in Roentgen Diagnosis*, L. C. de Leborgne (transl.). Montevideo, Impresora, Uruguay, S.A., 1953.
11. Lutterback, E. F.: Significance of mammography and xeroradiography in the early diagnosis of breast carcinoma. *Zentralbl Chir, 97*:713-719, 1972.
12. Mann, L. S., Japha, E. M., and Thomas, W., Jr.: Primary lymphoma of the breast. *Int Surg, 53*:108-114, 1970.
13. Martin, J. E.: Xeromammography—an improved diagnostic method. A review of 250 biopsied cases. *Am J Roentgenol Radium Ther Nucl Med, 117*:90-96, 1973.
14. Witten, D. M.: *The Breast*, Chicago, Yearbk. Med., 1969.
15. Wolfe, J. N.: *Mammography*. Springfield, Thomas, 1967.
16. Wolfe, J. N.: *Xeroradiography of the Breast*. Springfield, Thomas, 1972.
17. Wolfe, J. N.: Mammography. *Radiol Clin North Am, 12*:189-203, 1974.
18. Wolfe, J. N.: Mammography: errors in diagnosis. *Radiology, 87*:214-219, 1966.
19. Wolfe, J. N.: The prominent duct pattern as an indicator of cancer risk. *Oncology, 23*:149-158, 1969.
20. Wolfe, J. N.: Xerography of the breast. *Radiology, 91*:231-240, 1968.
21. Wolfe, J. N.: Xerography of the breast. *Cancer, 23*:791-796, 1969.
22. Wolfe, J. N.: Xeroradiography of the breast. *Oncology, 23*:113-119, 1969.

Index